Immunologic Considerations in Toxicology

Volume I

Editor

Raghubir P. Sharma
Professor of Toxicology
Utah State University
Logan, Utah

CRC Press, Inc.
Boca Raton, Florida

Library of Congress Cataloging in Publication Data

Main entry under title:

Immunologic considerations in toxicology.

Bibliography
Includes index.
Contents: v. 1. General mechanisms and environmental toxicants -- v. 2. Research methods and fish immunotoxicants.
1. Immunosuppression, 2. Toxicology.
3. Immunosuppressive agents. I. Sharma, Raghubir Prasad, 1940— . [DNLM: 1. Immunity.
2. Poisoning. QV 600 I33]
QR188.35.I46 615.9 80-39518
ISBN 0-8493-5271-1 (v. 1) AACR1
ISBN 0-8493-5272-X (v. 2)

Direct all inquiries to CRC Press, Inc., 2000 N.W. 24th Street, Boca Raton, Florida 33431.

International Standard Book Number 0-8493-5271-1 (v. 1)
International Standard Book Number 0-8493-5272-X (v. 2)

Library of Congress Card Number 80-39518
Printed in the United States

THE EDITOR

Raghubir P. Sharma is Professor of Toxicology in the Interdepartmental Toxicology Program at Utah State University and is affiliated with the Department of Animal, Dairy, and Veterinary Sciences.

He received his doctorate in Veterinary Medicine in 1959 from the University of Rajasthan, India, and a Ph.D. in 1968 from the University of Minnesota. During 1959-64, he worked as a veterinary clinician, instructor, and later as an assistant professor of pharmacology in his native country, India. From 1964 to 1969 he was a research fellow in the Department of Physiology and Pharmacology, at the School of Veterinary Medicine, University of Minnesota. Since 1969 he has been on the faculty of Utah State University, where he formerly was Assistant and later Associate Professor of Pharmacology and Toxicology. In 1976-77 he spent a sabbatical year at the Toxicology Research Laboratories of Dow Chemical Co., at Midland, Michigan. He is a naturalized U.S. citizen.

Dr. Sharma is a member of the Society of Toxicology, American Society for Pharmacology and Experimental Therapeutics, American Industrial Hygiene Association, American Veterinary Medical Association, American Society for Geochemistry and Health, American Association for the Advancement of Science, New York Academy of Sciences, and International Society for Biochemical Pharmacology. He is a Fellow of American College of Veterinary Toxicologists and a certified diplomate of the American Board of Veterinary Toxicology. He has been elected to the Societies of Sigma Xi and Phi Zeta. Dr. Sharma has served on several committees of various professional societies, and is currently Chairman of the Technical Committee of the Society of Toxicology (1980-81). He has been recipient of many research grants and contracts from the Public Health Service and several industrial foundations. He has been Director of the Interdepartmental Toxicology Program at Utah State University and is currently Associate Director of NIEHS Training grants in toxicology.

Dr. Sharma has authored or coauthored more than 100 scientific publications in the field of toxicology. His major research interests include biochemical mechanisms of toxicant effects, including those relating to the area of immunotoxicology.

CONTRIBUTORS

Jacques Banchereau, Ph.D.
Research Associate
School of Pharmacy
Chatenay Malabry, France

William A. Brindley, Ph.D.
Associate Professor Insecticide Toxicology
Department of Biology
Utah State University
Logan, Utah

Bernard Desoize, Ph.D.
Maitre-Assistant
Université de Reims
Faculté de Pharmacie
Reims, France

R. J. Kociba, D.V.M., Ph.D.
Group Leader
Pathology Section
Toxicology Research Laboratory
Dow Chemical Co.
Midland, Michigan

Loren D. Koller, D.V.M., Ph.D.
Associate Professor and Assistant Dean
School of Veterinary Medicine
University of Idaho
Moscow, Idaho

Colette Leger, Ph.D.
Research Associate
Unite de Toxicologie
Hospital Fernand Widal
Paris, France

Gabriel G. Nahas, M.D., Ph.D.
Professor
Department of Anesthesiology
Columbia University
College of Physicians and Surgeons
New York, New York

Steven G. Oberg, Ph.D.
Assistant Professor of Biology (Toxicology)
Utah State University
Logan, Utah

William Seinen, D.V.M., Ph.D.
Associate Professor
Working Group Pathology-Toxicology
Pathology and Pharmacology Toxicology Department
Faculty of Veterinary Sciences
State University Biltstraat
Utrecht, The Netherlands

Raghubir P. Sharma, D.V.M., Ph.D.
Professor of Toxicology
Utah State University
Logan, Utah

B. Singh, Ph.D.
Professor of Food Science and Technology
Alabama A and M University
Normal, Alabama

Joseph C. Street, Ph.D.
Professor Toxicology Program
Utah State University
Logan, Utah

J. G. Vos, D.V.M., Ph.D.
Director
Laboratory of Pathology
National Institute of Public Health
Bilthoven, The Netherlands

Philip G. Watanabe, Ph.D.
Group Leader
Molecular Toxicology
Toxicology Research Laboratory
Health and Environmental Research
The Dow Chemical Co.
Midland, Michigan

Maurice G. Zeeman, Ph.D.
Environmental Toxicologist
Food and Drug Administration
Bureau of Veterinary Medicine
Environmental Impact Staff
Rockville, Maryland

TABLE OF CONTENTS

VOLUME I

VOLUME II

Chapter 1

IMMUNOTOXICOLOGY: GENERAL CONSIDERATION

R. P. Sharma

TABLE OF CONTENTS

I. INTRODUCTION

The subdiscipline of toxicology dealing with the effects of chemicals on immune systems of animals and man is becoming referred to as *immunotoxicology*. The scope and content of immunotoxicology are not yet well recognized. The topic is usually considered within the realm of *immunopharmacology,* in which the therapeutic effects of chemicals on immune responses are considered, particularly in reference to the management of allergic diseases. By and large the drugs that are used in management of immune diseases are the well-known immunosuppressants. Recently, however, antianergic chemicals have been applied with variable success to stimulate the immune functions, particularly to increase the disease-free interval after surgical removal or radiotherapy of various types of tumors. Similarly, the effects of various environmental chemicals that have been investigated in the past were largely confined to their immunosuppressive potentials, and any other effects were considered either nonsignificant or of no toxicological consequence to the host.

It is obvious that the development of immunopharmacology or immunotoxicology has followed advances made in the science of immunology.* For a long time it has been known that certain drugs and chemicals influence the susceptibility of the host to infections and that this may be mediated through some effects on the immune system. The systematic investigations in the fields of immunopharmacology and immunotoxicology were made possible only after the steps involved in various immune mechanisms had been delineated and some understanding of their functions developed.

In a general sense both immune stimulation and suppression should be considered as abnormal reactions and perhaps toxic effects of chemicals. Although we do not know the exact significance of immune enhancement by chemicals, these may be considered as defensive or adaptive responses of the host. An insight into the mechanisms involved might prove valuable in understanding these proliferative responses.

II. WHY SHOULD IMMUNE EFFECTS BE STUDIED?

In a systematic toxicologic evaluation of new chemicals, the effects are generally considered on the basis of growth rate of animals or reduced function or weights or vital organs and their functions. Hematological parameters and the presence of any lesions in visceral organs are studied. In some cases, behavioral or neurological alterations are also investigated. It is generally considered that toxic effects of chemicals on immune responses have relevance when they can be adequately demonstrated at the exposure levels that prove to be nontoxic by traditional techniques of toxicity evaluation. This has proved to be true in some cases, e.g., treatment of experimental animals with mercury or lead can interfere with immune responses at dose levels that do not otherwise show toxic symptoms. In other cases, of course, the effects on immune functions may not appear until other pathological lesions are present and the effects may be considered as indirect ones.

Immune responses are important defense mechanisms for the host. Their impairment will allow an increased incidence of infection and thus may indirectly influence the survival of the individual or the species. In some cases the presence of mild infections may provide discomfort if the normal immune responses against them are delayed or decreased. Interference with normal immune reactions are therefore toxic, allowing

* The two journals devoted to these fields were recently published. One is by Pergamon Press, Oxford, and is the *International Journal of Immunopharmacology,* Edited by P. W. Mullen. The other one is by Marcel Dekker, New York, and is the *Journal of Immunopharmacology,* Edited by A. M. Reynard.

indirect interactions with the environment that may be partly biologic or antigenic in nature. The effects of chemicals, particularly of those that are present in the environment, upon immune systems should thus be evaluated.

Routine prophylactic immunization has had a remarkable impact on the control of infectious diseases. Vaccination against several of the notorious infectious agents has nearly wiped out their threat in most of the world, has effectively reduced mortality, and increased the average life expectancy. If chemicals inadvertantly interfere with the immunization process such interference may have serious consequences. In many cases, the individual may not be aware of the exposure to environmental chemicals that may be immunosuppressant. Investigation of the immunosuppressive potential of chemicals that people may accidently come in contact with is therefore desirable.

Chemicals may enter the body and affect specific target organs. Most of the chemicals we are concerned about are small molecules, not capable of mounting any antigenic responses. However, the damage to organs may cause a release of altered tissue components in the normal circulation that may be immunogenic. In some cases the chemicals or their metabolites are conjugated with normal or altered tissue components (e.g., proteins) and thus produce antigenic substances. This is a common mechanism of producing allergic conditions. Initial damage to organs and subsequent production of immune response against their tissue components may give rise to an autoimmune-phenomenon and often may be responsible for further damage in the host. Such haptenic potential of chemicals or the possibility of autoimmune-responses is worth investigating to assess the safety of chemicals.

The role of immune-surveillance in tumor survival has been proposed[1] and the thymus-dependent immune system may play a limited role in determining whether the initiated tumor will proliferate to a malignancy or not. Increased incidence of tumors has been shown in patients that were given immunosuppressive therapy after receiving a tissue or organ transplant. On the other hand, the "nude" mouse strain that lacks a thymus do not show an increased incidence of spontaneous tumors. Such conflicting evidence has not lent conviction to the argument that the immune system is important in retarding the development of the tumor from an incipient neoplasm. Nevertheless, increasing the effectiveness of immune responses has been reported to be useful in increasing the relapse-free interval after tumor destruction. The role of toxic chemicals in the incidence of neoplastic survival or remission may be important and should be evaluated. Further immunotoxicologic studies with potent chemicals will help solve the differences that have arisen in favor or against the immune-surveillance hypothesis. The investigations will perhaps provide additional insight into the effectiveness of various approaches in immunotherapy of neoplastic diseases.

An additional advantage of immunotoxicologic studies may be the investigations of basic biologic mechanisms. It is now well established that immune responses are mediated through highly selective and specific types of cells, i.e., T and B lymphocytes and macrophages. These cell types are capable of surviving in cultures and their responses can be manipulated by altering the culture conditions. Although the cells require a high degree of cooperation in vivo to bring about a coordinated immune effect, their functions have been selectively studied using in vitro systems. Use of various chemicals in these systems will help us understand the sites where these chemicals might be acting and thus provide valuable information on the nature of their chemical-biological interactions. We also know that cell functions are regulated by specific receptors on their surface membranes, which in turn regulate the replication of material in cells. Thus, immunotoxicologic studies can be valuable for investigating cellular models of the effects of reactive chemicals.

III. HOW CAN THE IMMUNOTOXICOLOGIC POTENTIAL BE EVALUATED?

There are a number of studies in the literature that deal with the testing of immune responses as affected by chemicals. The purpose of this treatise is to present an overview of the state of the art summarizing various reports and giving some additional newer information. Several investigators have used one or several tests in evaluating the effects on immune responses. It will be evident to the reader that all different functions of the immune system are not equally affected by chemicals. A chemical may show a profound effect on one parameter of the immunologic response whereas it may have no influence on other aspects while using different tests. That is, of course, not surprising since the immune response is a highly complex phenomenon and requires a number of steps to achieve the final response. On the other hand, there are distinct forms of immune responses, i.e., cellular vs. humoral types. It is, therefore, apparent that testing for immunologic potential is not simple, and a number of tests should be performed, particularly if some of the tests are proven to be negative.

A variety of techniques have been employed in immunotoxical testing. These range from the effect of infectious agents in the mortality of the test animal to the in vitro response of chemicals on the selective populations of immunocompetent cells. Various investigators have performed these tests but interlaboratory comparisons are very difficult to make because of variation in protocols employed. When conflicting reports are made by different workers using the same chemical, it is often impossible to say that this was really a variation on the response or was because of different technique. As more and more tests were developed in the field of immunology, they have been attempted by toxicologists, often without a clear comprehension of the principles involved. There is, therefore, a great need to provide a comprehensive review of these techniques for guidance of toxicologist.

A number of tests are usually needed to determine if a chemical indeed has a biologically important effect on immune functions, but usually these tests can be performed easily and can be readily incorporated in chronic toxicity testing. More elaborate testing will be necessary only if a potential effect is indicated. Information in Volume II, Chapters 5 and 6 will provide some insight into the approaches for the testing for immunotoxicological effects.

It is not sufficient to say that a chemical has an effect on the immune response as, for example, that it is immunosuppressive. It is desirable in many cases to elucidate the exact location of action on the immune function. If the mechanism is known, the potential of the chemical, particularly at low level exposures, can be ascertained with more objectivity. It will also be possible to relate the in vitro findings to those observed in vivo. At a future time then it might be possible to propose a more specific and brief protocol for studying new chemicals. At present there is little information on the cellular or molecular level at which the chemicals cause their effect on the immune system.

The importance of the immunotoxicologic potential has been recently emphasized. Professional organizations and regulatory agencies have shown an increased interest in the possibility of immunotoxicologic testing and toxicological roles of chemicals in immune functions.* It is likely that the research and emphasis in this new discipline will

* During 1978, several conferences emphasizing immunotoxicology and related aspects were held. Some of these were (1) Gordon Conference on Toxicology and Safety Evaluation, Meridan, N.H. (2) N.Y. Acad. Sci., International Conference on Halogenated Hydrocarbons, New York, and (3), Inadvertant Modification of Immune Responses, FDA Symposium, Annapolis, MD.

increase in the future as more information becomes available and there is an increased awareness to this problem which has received very little attention in the past.

Some obvious precautions will be indicated in studies undertaken to determine effects on immune responses. As suggested earlier, a number of tests can be incorporated in the chronic toxicity testing schedule. But the selection of dose levels should be highly important. Large doses of chemicals that cause other pathologic effects or decreases in organ weights are likely to show immunotoxicologic effects regardless whether a chemical has a direct effect on the immune system or not. A cytotoxic effect of the chemical at a large dose or the incidence of organ damage may be responsible for a subsequent effect on host immune responses.

It has been reported that stress on animals can alter their immune functions. Incorporation of a large dose of a chemical in the dietary regimen may cause stress or a deficiency of essential nutrients and thus alter the metabolism of the animal. Stress has been shown to alter the incidence of neoplastic survival. It is highly likely that this action may be mediated through an early effect on the immune system.

As more and more chemicals are employed in immunotoxicolgic studies and their mechanisms are elucidated, this may give rise to information that may further help to understand immune mechanisms. Various mitogenic agents that are used in lymphocyte cultures, for example, have proved highly valuable. A number of chemicals similarly have mitogenic properties (see Volume II, Chapter 7) and can be used in dissecting the immune mechanisms at various steps. This may also lead to a better appreciation of the receptor molecules, especially if the structural requirements for agonists or antagonists are established in immune cells.

IV. CHEMICALS IMPORTANT FOR IMMUNOTOXICOLOGIC EVALUATIONS

The need to evaluate chemicals to which the exposure is either inadvertant or unavoidable should be emphasized. In an industrial environment, for example, exposure of workers to traces of chemicals is almost inevitable. Although consumers are only concerned with the final product, industrial workers have to deal with a number of highly reactive starting materials or their intermediates. An illustration in case may be the plastic industry which has been elaborated on in Chapter 8. Plastics are polymerized chemicals and there is little danger from monomeric materials during the use of the final products. In the manufacturing process, however, industrial workers may come in contact with a number of chemicals, some of which do have immunotoxicologic properties. As indicated later, a number of dermatoses or other allergic problems are related to immunologic mechanisms. Even if the environmental concentrations of these chemicals are sufficiently lowered, the contact is repetitive and often lasts for several years. Moreover, there is rarely a dose-response relationship between the immunologic effects and the causative chemicals. A thorough evaluation of chemicals that may be present in the industrial environment is thus highly desirable.

Another class of chemicals that poses a threat of repeated exposure includes food additives and preservatives. It is possible that even natural products in foods may have immunotoxicologic properties (see Chapter 11). Little attention has been given to these food additives with regards to their potential as immunosuppressants. Some of these have been investigated but more need to be studied since the efforts required for immunotoxicologic testing are far less than those for other chronic tests that are desired, e.g., determining carcinogenic potential. Food constituents are additionally important for determining their toxic effects on the immune system since such effects can alter the response of organisms to various toxins that are sometimes encountered in food products.

Various air and water contaminants also deserve attention in immunologic testing since the exposure to these can also be prolonged. Very little work has been done on local immune mechanisms dealing with inhaled pollutants, both gaseous and particulate. Exposing animals to chemicals in inhalation chambers may or may not produce any effect on their splenic or thymic functions, but it is likely that the lung immune responses will be affected since the insult is direct and in the case of particulate material the exposure concentration in local tissues in the pulmonary system may be relatively high. Studies dealing with local defense systems of the body, i.e., lung macrophage and lymphatics for inhaled chemicals and the gut associated immune responses for orally ingested chemicals, should be conducted.

There are several other environmental pollutants that have gained attention in recent years. Some of these are indeed immunotoxic. Several reports on PCB and PBB indicate that these chemicals have some effect on immune mechanisms. These chemicals have been incorporated in our food chain and have already gained access to the human body before anything could be done. A very potent immunotoxic agent, TCDD, is another example of an environmental pollutant of interest in this regard. Contamination of soil and other components of the environment through the use of materials in which it was a contaminant, and the possibility of an industrial accident like the one in Seveso, Italy, has raised serious questions about the health hazards of TCDD.[2] A review of its immunotoxicologic investigations is presented in Chapter 9.

V. ORGANIZATION OF THE CURRENT VOLUMES

The information in these two volumes is presented in four parts that deal with related but slightly different aspects of immunotoxicology. The following four chapters deal with the basic review of immunological concepts. Readers familiar with this discipline will find it too elementary or even superficial. The purpose is primarily to familiarize toxicologists, who may have little background in the field of immunology with immunological functions. The details of various aspects are not included for the sake of simplicity. Newer concepts that have not fully been accepted or the ones that are controversial are purposefully avoided. Some of the material in these chapters is arranged to provide a transition to other parts of the book and hence the emphasis on each part is not necessarily equal.

The second part consists of reviews dealing with the status of immunotoxicological evaluations. The topics are selected to include major environmental contaminants and studies conducted with selected chemicals. The purpose of these reviews is not necessarily to provide a comprehensive compilation of the literature but to present the state of the art as it deals with each of the topics discussed. It will be obvious that the immunotoxicologic evaluation has a long ways to go before a consensus on the health hazards of a contaminant can be reached.

The third part (in Volume II) contains selected research reports in the area of immunotoxicology. These deal with some of the problems of current interest and provide an insight into new approaches that are being employed. One of the contributions involves the possible evaluation of a neurotoxic organophosphate and whether or not it produces its effects via autoimmunologic mechanisms.

The final and fourth part in the second volume includes a few chapters dealing with the models of testing and some of the techniques that have been found useful in this field. Only the procedures that are simple enough and can be easily adopted by toxicology laboratories are included here. Because of the continuing advances in the field of immunology, more and more techniques are likely to become available in the future. When the steps involved in immunologic regulation are well understood, newer methods can be used to investigate the mechanisms of immunotoxicologic actions.

A glossary of the selected terms used in this book is provided at the end. This may be useful for readers with little familiarity with immunological literature.

REFERENCES

1. **Burnet, F. M.,** The concept of immunological surveillance, *Prog. Exp. Tumor Res.*, 13, 1, 1970.
2. **Reggiani, G.,** Medical problems raised by TCDD contamination in Seveso, Italy, *Arch. Toxicol.*, 40, 161, 1978.

Chapter 2

IMMUNITY AND THE IMMUNE SYSTEM

R. P. Sharma

TABLE OF CONTENTS

I. INTRODUCTION

Most organisms have defense mechanisms that protect them from external invaders of biological origin. In higher organisms this function is carried out by a highly developed and complex immune system. The immune system responds to various macromolecules that are termed *antigenic,* and which are generally the components of invading biological organisms. Proteins and other large biological molecules are antigenic in nature in the sense that an immunologic defense can be mounted against them. Many small molecules, although not antigenic by themselves, can elicit specific immune reactivity because they may be linked to other large molecules like proteins and hence become antigenic. Such small molecules thus conjugated to proteins are termed *hapten.*

Immune reactions can be produced against any large molecule that is foreign to the host, including the cellular components of an allogeneic organism. The reactions are sometimes elicited in response to an altered host tissue protein, as in the case of damage or organs or tissues, leading to an autoimmune reaction. The presence of a macromolecule at places where it is not supposed to be can also initiate an immune response. For example, the immune response can be mounted against the nervous tissue from an otherwise compatible donor if the tissue is injected systemically.

II. THE LYMPHATIC SYSTEM

It is now well established that the lymphatic system is the main unit of immune responses, together with the macrophages and the reticuloendothelial system present in many organs. The lymphatic system consists of primary lymphatic organs (where differentiation of lymphocytes occurs, i.e., thymus and bursa or its mammalian equivalent — fetal liver and later bone marrow) and secondary or peripheral organs through which the lymphocytes migrate. The secondary organs include the spleen and lymph nodes, as well as peritoneal cavity and lymphatic ducts. The lymphatic ducts connect various lymphoid organs with general circulation. Birds do not have well defined lymph nodes and the primary lymphoid organs are connected to circulation by lymphatic ducts. Various parenchymatous organs in birds have a diffuse lymphatic channel system.

The detailed anatomical structures of various lymphoid organs have been described elsewhere.[1] The basic unit of the lymphatic system are lymphocytes present both in peripheral circulation and different lymphoid organs. These cells along with other differential cells such as plasma cells, macrophages, polymorphonuclear (PMN) leukocytes and blast cells are involved in the responses that collectively characterize the immune function.

Like other cells of the hematopoietic system the different immunocytes are produced in the bone marrow. The stem cells, which originate in the bone marrow and are further differentiated into various hematologic components, cannot be distinguished from each other. The precursors of lymphocytes originate in the bone marrow of adults or in the fetal liver (or yolk sac in birds) in the prenatal organism. They then migrate either to thymus or the bursa of Fabricius or its mammalian equivalent. Following the differentiation in the primary lymphoid organs, the immunocompetent cells leave their differentiating organs and do not return there in appreciable numbers. A number of stem cells produced in the bone marrow in adult mammals, however, acquire surface immunoglobulins and migrate to the spleen, the others normally homing to various lymph nodes.[2]

In thymic cortex the residential cells undergo constant divisions with a complete turnover of cells in 3-4 days.[3] Only a very small fraction of these, however, leave the organ to enter circulation. Others are destroyed in the thymus itself. In lymph nodes, a small number of cells are derived from cell division in the node itself. The rest of them entering from the circulating pool, mostly from blood and a small fraction through efferent lymphatic channels.[4] In most mammalian species, the lymphocytes leave the lymph node via efferent channels and enter the circulation through the thoracic duct. Although both B and T lymphocytes (bursa and thymus, respectively) enter the lymph node together, the B cells preferentially migrate towards the cortex and form the germinal centers. The T cells remain primarily in the paracortical area. Plasma cells, however, are found generally in the medullary region suggesting that the B cells have to migrate through a T cell-dependent area. The transit time of T lymphocytes from circulation through the lymph node and back to the thoracic duct has been estimated to be 18-24 hr. B cells have a slightly longer retention time in lymph nodes, approximately 30 hr. The longer transit time of B cells is not dependent on their splenic retention.[5] Rabbits and sheep have virtually no B cells in their peripheral circulation.[6]

In spleen both B and T cells enter from the arterial circulation in the periarterial lymphatic zone and migrate peripherally.[6] B lymphocytes accumulate to form germinal centers that do not have T cells. Both B and T cells leave the spleen via the marginal zone channels leading to the red pulp, and from there may leave this organ via splenic vein.

III. HUMORAL VS. CELLULAR IMMUNITY

It has now been well recognized that two separate types of immune responses can be mounted against antigenic invaders and the two mechanisms are mediated through different populations of lymphocytes. The humoral mechanisms, mediated through the production of antigen-specific antibodies, are carried out by B lymphocytes. B cells are named after the discovery that the bursa of Fabricius in chicken was responsible for differentiating cells involved in the production of antibodies.[7] The cell-mediated immunity depends on T cells which are thymus-dependent, and can be abolished by thymic irradiation or neonatal thymectomy. The cellular immune responses are absent in athymic animals, e.g., nude mice. Although the two mechanisms are largely different, the different types of cells cooperate with each other. For example, T cells are important in influencing the ultimate expression of humoral immunity. A simplified diagrammatic representation of lymphocyte differentiation is presented in Figure 1. The description of the two types of immune reactions is further elaborated in the chapters that follow.

IV. B AND T LYMPHOCYTES

Differentiation of primordial stem cells into functional B and T lymphocytes is described later in Chapters 3 and 4. Some of the structural and functional differences between the two will be mentioned here. Both B and T cells are structurally indistinguishable from each other in their size and shape when observed under a conventional microscope. Scanning electron microscopy, however, has provided valuable distinguishing features in these two types of cells.

Figure 2 illustrates a murine B lymphocyte as it appears under a scanning electron microscope. B cell surfaces are covered with microvilli or fingerlike projections, which are rare or scanty on the T cells. The surfaces of the two types of cells are functionally different as they contain molecules for different types of receptors. T lymphocytes from certain inbred mice strains (C3H, CBA), for example, contain lymphocyte alloantigens (called θ or thy 1 antigen) on their surface, while these antigens are absent on B cells. These alloantigens are present on other cells such as those of brain, skin and fibroblasts. Anti-θ sera can be prepared to neutralize the functional characters of T lymphocytes and for their recognition. Another series of alloantigens called ly alloantigens (Ly 1, 2,

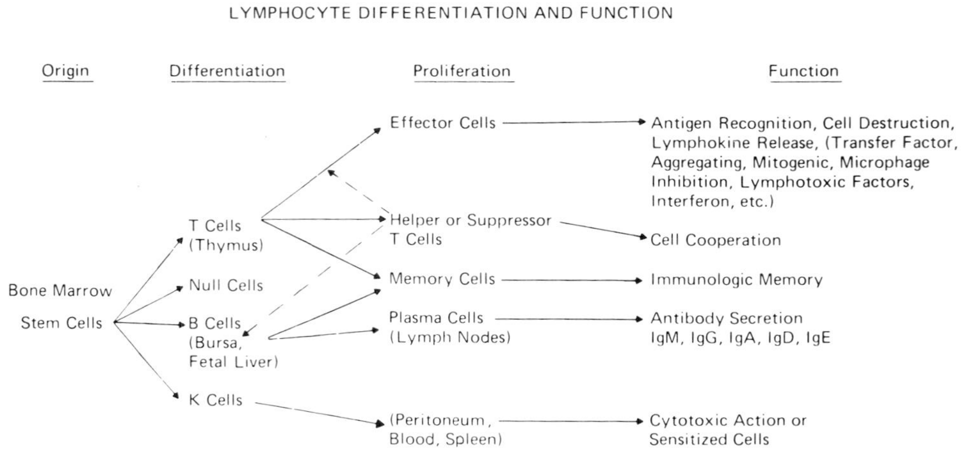

FIGURE 1. A simplified scheme of differentiation of lymphocytes to their subpopulations along with major functions.

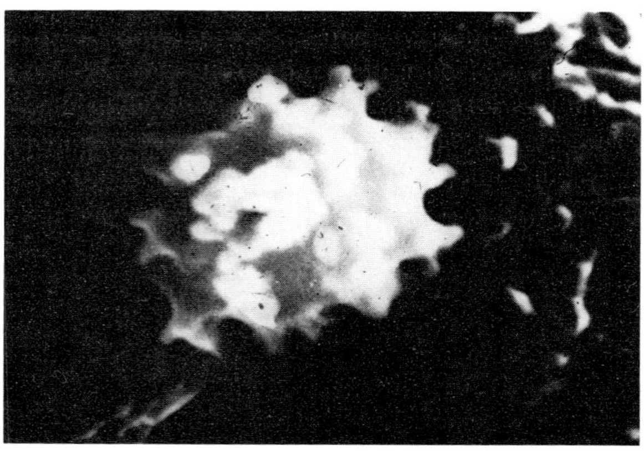

FIGURE 2. Scanning electron micrograph of a murine lymphocyte. The projections on the surface are typical of B cells (photograph courtesy of Lyla Wagley, Utah State University).

3, and 5) are restricted to T lymphocyte surfaces but Ly 4 is present both on T and B cells. T cells can be distinguished in a population by the heterosera prepared against thymus or brain (heteroantigens) which can be made specific by absorption with B cells.[9] Similarly, B cell specific antisera can be prepared from the homogeneous population of B cells, such as from human chronic lymphocytic leukemia.

V. SURFACE RECEPTORS ON LYMPHOCYTES

In addition to the alloantigens present on lymphocyte surfaces as mentioned above, there are other types of receptors that distinguish the two cell populations. T lymphocytes of certain species contain specific receptors for erythrocytes of other species. For example, T cells from man and pig have receptors for sheep enythrocytes, whereas guinea pig T cells have those for rabbit red blood cells.[10] These receptors provide an easy approach for differentiating the T lymphocytes by the technique of rosette formation. If human lymphocytes are gently mixed with sheep erythrocytes and centrifuged, the T cells will appear under a microscope as a rosette of erythrocytes aggregated around the cells. These heterologous erythrocyte receptors are different from the antigen-receptors and do not require the presence of immunoglobulin on T cell surface. The lymphocytes involved in humoral immunity (B cells) have surface receptors for active fixed complement (C3b).[11] Red cells coated with such complement will form rosettes with B cells and also with macrophages or other cells (PMN leukocytes, platelets). Primate erythrocytes have similar receptors. The lymphoid cells other than T cells also have receptors for the Fc portion of IgG (See Chapter 3). These receptors can play a valuable role in the techniques used for characterizing different types of cells. A number of lymphocytes have specific receptors for viruses, specific antigens and macromolecules that elicit the mitogenic transformation of immune competent cells.

VI. RESPONSIVENESS OF LYMPHOCYTES AGAINST MITOGENS

In the body the specific subpopulations of B or T lymphocytes undergo clonal division when there is an antigen challenge. This division is preceded by the formation of blast cells that ultimately divide into clones. The sensitized cells often respond to a subsequent challenge of the same antigen at an amplified level. The process of cell division is simulated in an in vitro system if the lymphocytes sensitized in vivo are treated with the same antigen in a culture. A similar phenomenon is observed when the lymphocytes are incubated in the presence of certain lectins derived from plants or similar macromolecules. Different populations of cells appear to have different types of receptors that can be distinguished by the mitogenic stimulation in cultures. The molecules that cause the transformation of lymphocytes are mitogens or blastogens, and although some of these bind with both types of cells, they can be selective in blast formation in lymphocyte subpopulations.

The response of lymphocytes to different mitogens has been used to evaluate the functional ability of lymphocytes or their subpopulations. It has also provided us with a diagnostic tool for identifying certain diseases. Table 1 includes a listing of selected mitogens, their sources and the cells that are affected. Although the exact implications of mitogenic stimulation are not well understood, lymphocyte transformation techniques have been employed in immunotoxicological assessment of chemicals and drugs.

VII. GENERAL FACTORS INFLUENCING IMMUNE RESPONSES

A variety of physiological and environmental factors are known to cause modifications of the immune reactions. Some of these may be hormonal factors, i.e., thymosin, that is required for the maturation of thymocytes. Steroid hormones and their various synthetic analogs have immunosuppressant properties. A number of drugs have been used both to cause suppression of immune reactions and also to stimulate the responses if they were suppressed. Use of adjuvant materials (e.g., bacterial cell wall preparations) in conjunction with various antigens has been recognized to stimulate the immunity against the antigen used. Some of these factors have been discussed below.

A soluble product derived from the thymus, called thymosin, has been shown to affect the maturation of thymocytes.[12] The injection of thymus does not always, however, reverse the effects of neonatal thymectomy, although the passage of soluble factors from thymus implants within a diffusion chamber that does not allow migration of living cells repairs the immunological defects produced by thymectomy. The cells devoid of the thy antigen can be converted to competent thymic cells when incubated with the thymus extracts, even though the extract does not contain any thy antigen.

Table 1
MITOGENIC AGENTS USED FOR LYMPHOCYTE PROLIFERATION IN CELL CULTURES

Mitogen (Source)	Abbreviation	General use or target cells
Phytohemagglutinin *Phaseolus vulgaris*	PHA	Indicative of T cell function. Mature thymus cells are more responsive than immature ones.
Concanavalin A *Canavalis ensiformis*	Con A	Indicative of immature T cell reactivity.
Pokeweed mitogen *Phytolocca americana*	PWM	Nonspecific lymphocyte stimulant. Generally used to indicate B cell responsiveness.
Bacterial Lipopolysaccharide *Escherichia coli*	LPS	Specific for B cell response.
Purified protein derivative *Mycobacterium tuberculosis*	PPD	Stimulates B cells but also a T cell stimulant in tuberculin sensitized individuals or animals.
Specific antigen or hapten	—	Can be employed to evaluate the specific response, e.g., in case of allergy.
Lymphokines *Mixed cell cultures*	MLC	To evaluate the general responsiveness of lymphocytes as stimulated by the presence of allogeneic cells. Process believed to be macrophage dependent.

Corticosteroids have long been recognized as possessing lympholytic properties. Natural adrenocorticosteroids as well as their synthetic analogs reduce the size and lymphoid contents of the lymph nodes and spleen although they do not produce any affect on proliferating stem cells of bone marrow.[13] The mechanism of action of these chemicals is not well understood, but they are believed to interfere with the cell cycle of activated lymphocytes. Both cellular and humoral immune responses are suppressed by the glucocorticoids; the effects may be different at different stages of cell differentiation. These chemicals have gained popularity in their clinical use as immunosuppressants in conditions like organ transplant or in the management of autoimmune diseases.

Different types of stress are known to alter the individual's sensitivity to infection. Adverse physical stimuli cause a physiological stress exemplified by the general adaptation syndrome. Among the somatic characteristics of the general adaptation syndrome are included hypertrophy of the adrenal cortex and atrophy of lymphatic tissue.[14] Environmental stress has been shown to cause an increase in the amount of circulating glucocorticoids.

A number of other cytotoxic alkylating agents, e.g., 6-mercaptopurine, cyclophosphamide, are clinically used as immunosuppressants in conjunction with the glucocorticoids.[13] These chemicals are potent inhibitors of protein synthesis and are employed in autoimmune disorders or in organ transplantation patients to prevent the graft rejection. The environmental chemicals that are of concern in immunotoxicology are nowhere similar to these chemicals in their potency.

A potent alkaline phosphate inhibitor, levamisole, has been used as an immunostimulant or anti-anergic agent in man and experimental animals. It has been investigated for its possible therapeutic applications in diseases associated with the impairment of cellular immunity. In cancer patients, treatment with levamisole after surgery or radiation therapy, either alone or in conjunction with other antimetabolites, has been known to prolong the disease-free interval.[15] In an experimental situation, this chemical promotes the rejection of isograft in mice and produces an enhancement of the delayed type hypersensitivity.[16] Addition of levamisole to lymphocyte cultures did not alter the blast formation in the presence or absence of phytohemagglutinin.[17] It has been proposed that the efficacy of levamisole in stimulating immune responses is greater in individuals that have depressed immune functions.

Individuals and animals can be made unresponsive to an antigenic stimulation. This phenomenon has been referred to as immunotolerance or immune paralysis. Generalized immune tolerance may occur by genetic defects or may be produced by the destruction or elimination of primary lymphoid organs. Damage to the lymphatic system by X-rays or immunotherapy leads to a general immunotolerance. Specific immunotolerance can be produced either by antigens or antibodies to the antigen receptors on the immunocompetent cells. The agents that lead to immunotolerance are called tolerogens and the phenomenon is often dose-dependent.[1] Immunologic unresponsiveness can be exhibited to a different antigen after a challenge with another antigen; this usually persists for several days after the first challenge.[18] Several models of specific immunotolerance production by antigens and antibodies have been proposed.[19] The exact mechanism of tolerance is not well understood. It perhaps involves several different pathways both at the specific cellular level and also at the level of the antigen, that produces immune effects.

VIII. GENERAL APPROACHES IN STUDYING THE EFFECTS OF CHEMICALS ON IMMUNE RESPONSES

As would become evident after a quick review of the chapters that follow in this treatise, there is no single or simple test that can be used for the evaluation of either immunosuppressive or immune-enhancing effects of test chemicals. Various plans and models proposed by different workers are elaborated in Volume II, Chapters 5 and 6. Based on the types of tests employed in different studies, the various approaches that are used in immunological testing are summarized in Tables 2-5. Table 2 consists of a list of tests that have been used in the evaluation of generalized immune responses by environmental chemicals. Specific tests employed for the testing of humoral and cell-mediated immunity are indicated in Tables 3 and 4, respectively. The picture is not complete until the important interacting cells in various immune functions, i.e., macrophages, are also considered. The macrophages play an important role both in humoral and cellular immune responses by cooperating with selective immunocytes. Little emphasis has been placed on studying these cells in various immunotoxicologic evaluations. The awareness of the role of macrophages in immunotoxicology is becoming more important and interesting. Some of the tests that have been used in the toxicological testing and included later in this book are listed in Table 5. Undoubtedly more tests of different kinds have been performed and will be added to these lists as more data on immunologic testing becomes available and more is known about the immunologic mechanisms governing the activities of various cells and their subpopulations.

In vitro tests using heterogeneous mixtures of cells or their isolated subpopulations are becoming more useful. In many cases the reactivity of specific cells to surface–acting agents can be readily evaluated in vitro by using the mitogens mentioned in Table 1. Direct effects of chemicals can be evaluated by their addition to cultures but should be viewed with caution. A number of chemicals decrease the response of lymphocytes to blastogenic agents by virtue of being cytotoxic. On the other hand, some chemicals may have nonspecific mitogenic properties themselves. Interaction of chemicals with mitogens in the medium may modify their function. Similar effects can be produced if the interfering molecules in the medium such as specific fractions of serum proteins are neutralized or altered by the presence of test chemicals.

Table 2
GENERAL TESTS EMPLOYED FOR IMMUNOTOXICOLOGY EVALUATION OF ENVIRONMENTAL CHEMICALS

Test	Chemicals tested	Chapter(s) and Volume
Weights of lymphatic organs (thymus, spleen, lymph nodes)	Various	6, 9, 10 (Volume I), 6 (Volume II)
Lesions or alterations in lymphatic organs	TCDD, TOTP pesticides	6, 9, 10 (Volume I), 4 (Volume II)
Peripheral lymphocyte counts — total and relative to other leucocytes	Various	6, 7, 9, 10, 12 (Volume I)
Presence of immune complex	Vinyl chloride	8 (Volume I)
Infectivity of challenge with mixed antigens	Various	6—10 (Volume I)
Survival of transplanted tumors or cells	Various	9 (Volume I), 5 (Volume II)
Epidemiological Survey	TCDD	9 (Volume I)
Lymphocyte transformation	Various	7—10, (Volume I), 2, 3, 7, (Volume II)

Table 3
TESTS FOR EVALUATING HUMORAL IMMUNITY

Test employed	Chemical tested	Chapter(s) and Volume
Measurements of globulins, total or specific	Various	6—12 (Volume I), 1, 4, 5, 8 (Volume II)
Complement levels	Vinyl chloride	8 (Volume I)
Specific antibody titers (thymus independent antigens)	Various	6—10, 12, (Volume I), 1 (Volume II)
Antibody forming cells in spleen or lymph nodes. (plaque-assay)	Pesticides, metals	6, 7 (Volume I)
Fluorescence visualization of plasma cells in lymphatic organs	Pesticides PCB	6 (Volume I)
Markers for B lymphocytes	Various	2, 3, 5 (Volume II)
Specific B cell mitogens	Pesticides, metals cannabinoids, drugs	6, 7, (Volume I), 2, 3, 5, 7 (Volume II)

Table 4
TESTS FOR EVALUATING CELL MEDIATED IMMUNITY

Test employed	Chemicals tested	Chapter(s) and Volume
Delayed hypersensitivity (skin reactivity to PPD)	Various	6, 7, 9, (Volume I), 4 (Volume II)
Adjuvant induced arthritis	Drugs	—
Tail-graft survival	TCDD	9 (Volume I)
Host-vs.-Graft assay	TCDD	9 (Volume I), 5 (Volume II)
Response to thymus-dependent antigens	Various	9, 10, (Volume I), 5 (Volume II)
T cell mitogens	Various	6—10, 12 (Volume I), 1—3, 5, 7 (Volume II)
T cell markers, Rosette formation	Various	7 (Volume I), 5 (Volume II)
Tests for lymphokines	Various	5 (Volume II)

Table 5
MACROPHAGE TESTS USED IN IMMUNOTOXICOLOGIC EVALUATION

Test employed	Chemicals tested	Chapter(s) and Volume
Accumulation of bacteria in lymphatic organs	TCDD	9 (Volume I)
Nonspecific phagocytosis	Metals, TCDD	7, 9 (Volume I)
Metabolic activity of phagocytes (nitro-blue tetrazolium reduction)	TCDD	9 (Volume I)
Enzyme assay in macrophage system	Pesticides, others	6, 7 (Volume I), 5 (Volume II)

Lymphocyte cultures in vitro are valuable when carried out after administering the test chemicals to the animals and then looking for the mitogenic responsiveness of cells harvested from major lymphatic organs. In this case the test chemical can be transformed in the body if its action is dependent on the formation of reactive metabolite. Direct addition of metabolizing systems (i.e., mixed function oxidases of liver microsomal systems) have not been of value since their presence may modify lymphocyte transformation in vitro. At the same time the chemicals modifying the immunologic mechanisms indirectly, i.e., through alteration of other systems like steroid levels, can be suitably evaluated by in vivo administration of chemicals. Various immunotolerant mechanisms require specific T suppressor cells or macrophages at other locations than from where the lymphocytes are harvested, or may involve autoimmunologic responses through haptenic conjugations and these can be detected only by the administration of test chemicals in the intact animal.

REFERENCES

1. **Sell, S. Ed.,** *Immunology, Immunopathology and Immunity,* 2nd ed., Harper and Row, New York, 1975, 384.
2. **Osmond, D. G. and Nossal, G. J. V.,** Differentiation of Lymphocytes in mouse bone marrow. I. Quantitative autoradiographic studies of antiglobulin binding by lymphocytes in bone marrow and lymphoid tissues, *Cell Immunol.,* 13, 117, 1974.
3. **Miller, J. R. A. P. and Osoba, D.,** Current concepts of the immunological function of the thymus. *Physiol. Rev.,* 47, 437, 1967.
4. **Hall, J. G. and Morris, B. J.,** The origin of the cells in the efferent lymph from a single lymph node, *J. Exp. Med.,* 121, 901, 1965.
5. **Ford, W. L.,** Lymphocyte migration and immune responses, *Prog. Allergy,* 19, 1, 1975.
6. **McConnell, I.,** Structure and function of Lymphoid tissue, in, *The Immune System,* Hobart, M. J. and McConnell, I., Eds., *Blackwell Scientific,* Oxford, 1975.
7. **Glick, B., Chang, T. S., and Japp, R. G.,** The bursa of Fabricius and antibody production, *Poult. Sci.,* 35, 224, 1956.
8. **Raff, M. C.,** Surface antigenic markers for distinguishing T and B lymphocytes in mice, *Transplant Rev.,* 6, 52, 1971.
9. **Golub, E. S.,** Brain-associated θ antigen: reactivity of rabbit anti-mouse brain with mouse lymphoid cells, *Cell Immunol.,* 2, 353, 1971.
10. **McConnell, I.,** T and B lymphocytes, in, *The Immune System* Hobart, M. J. and McConnell, I., Eds., *Blackwell Scientific,* Oxford, 1975.
11. **Ross, G. D., Polley, M. J., Rabellino, E. M., and Grey, H. M.,** Two different complement receptors on human lymphocytes. One specific for C3b and one for C3b inactivator-cleaved C3b, *J. Exp. Med.,* 138, 798, 1973.

12. **Goldstein, A. L. and White, A.,** Thymosin and other thymic hormones: Their nature and roles in the thymic dependency in immunological phenomenon, in, *Contemporary Topics in Immunology,* Vol 2. Davis, A. J. S. and Carter, R. L., Eds., Plenum Press, New York, 1973, 339.
13. **Salmon, S. E.,** Drugs and the immune system, in, *Review of Medical Pharmacology,* Meyers, F. J., Jawetz, E., and Goldfien, A., Eds., Lange, 446, 1970.
14. **Thaxton, P. and Briggs, D. M.,** Effect of immobilization and formaldehyde on immunological responsiveness in young chickens, *Poultry Sci.,* 51, 342, 1972.
15. **Wilkins, S. A. and Olkowski, Z. L.,** Immunocompetence of cancer patients treated with levamisole, *Cancer (Philadelphia),* 39, 487, 1977.
16. **Renoux, G., Renoux, M., Teller, M. N., McMahon, S., and Guillaumin, J. M.,** Potentiation of T cell mediated immunity by levamisole, *Clin. Exp. Immunol.,* 25, 288, 1976.
17. **Merryman, P. and Jaffe, I. A.,** Effect of levamisole on phytohemagglutinin-stimulated human lymphocytes, *Biochem. Pharmacol.,* 26, 1358, 1977.
18. **Weigle, W. O.,** Recent observations and concepts in immunological unresponsiveness and autoimmunity, *Clin. Exp. Immunol.,* 9, 537, 1971.
19. **Rowley, D. A., Fitch, F. W., Stuart, F. P., Köhler, H., and Cosenza, H.,** Specific suppression of immune responses, *Science,* 181, 1133, 1973.

Chapter 3

HUMORAL IMMUNITY

L. D. Koller

TABLE OF CONTENTS

I. ORIGIN AND DIFFERENTIATION OF B LYMPHOCYTES

B lymphocytes arise from hematopoietic stem cells which originate in the yolk sac of the avian and mammalian embryo. Stem cells are multipotential and can differentiate into any of the mature lymphoid or myeloid types. It is presumed that multipotential stem cells give rise to progenator stem cells that are restricted in their differentiating capacity thereby producing specific blood cells such as T or B lymphocytes.[1]

Hematopoietic derived B cells of the chicken lodge in the bursa of Fabricius where they subsequently differentiate and mature within follicles for the production and secretion of immunoglobulins.[2] Mammals lack a bursa and an analogous organ has not been defined. It is not known where B cell precursors become committed to synthesize immunoglobulins in mammals even though stem cells that can mature into B lymphocytes have been identified in fetal liver[3] and bone marrow.[4] Various gastrointestinal lymphoid tissues have also been suggested as the mammalian bursal equivalents but little evidence has been established that any of these tissues contribute in B lymphocyte maturation.

Lymphocytes are separated into T and B cells on basis of ontogeny, surface membrane markers, and functions. T and B lymphocytes differ in several respects including size, density, surface charge, adherence properties, surface membrane markers, migration patterns, tissue distribution and turnover rates.[5] B lymphocytes can be identified and separated from T lymphocytes by utilizing these properties.

There are three categories of B lymphocytes,[6] immature (pre–virgin) B cells, virgin B cells, and memory B cells. Immature B lymphocytes do not have surface immunoglobulin and are usually large cells. Immature B cells cannot be immunized but are sensitive to tolerogenesis. Virgin B lymphocytes are small, noncirculating cells concentrated in solid tissue. They have a rapid turnover rate, low surface charge, monovalent receptors, and are continually produced in adult bone marrow from rapidly dividing medium and large lympocyte precursors.[5,6,7] The nondividing virgin lymphocytes acquire detectable immunoglobulin receptors (IgM) through maturation. Virgin B lymphocytes, when stimulated by antigen, become activated and differentiate into effector cells (plasma cells which secrete antibody) and memory B cells. The memory cells are long–lived small lymphocytes which recirculate and are concentrated in thoracic duct lymph. They have a high surface charge, slow turnover rate, and possess multivalent receptors which are primarily IgG.

To reiterate B cell ontogeny, stem cells and precursor B cells repopulate antigen–sensitive B lymphocytes as required from bone marrow which is the primary site of continuous production and differentiation of immunoglobulin bearing small lymphocytes. These cells interact with each other and antigen to trigger differentiation which gives rise to effector cells or memory B cells. The effector cells produce and secrete antibody while the memory cells are responsible primarily for secondary responses.

For clinical and experimental purposes, B cells are recognized by surface receptors. B lymphocytes bear membrane–associated immunoglobulin which can be easily detected by using fluorescein-conjugated anti-immunoglobulin.[8] B cells also have surface receptors for the activated third component (C3 receptor) of complement.[9] A procedure used to detect B cells involves the binding of sheep erythrocytes absorbed with antibody and complement (EAC complexes) to the C3 receptor on B cells to form rosettes.[10] Receptors for the Fc portions of IgG molecules are also present on B lymphocytes and are demonstrated by the EA (sheep erythrocytes-antibody) assay.[11] Macrophages also have C and Fc receptors while some T lymphocytes bear Fc receptors. It is possible that B lymphocytes may also have receptors for macrophages and T cell factors.

II. STRUCTURE AND FUNCTION OF IMMUNOGLOBULINS

Immunoglobulins (antibodies) are a group of glycoproteins closely related by structure and function. Five major classes of immunoglobulins (IgM, IgG, IgA, IgE, and IgD) have been identified on the basis of their physical, chemical, and antigenic properties.[2]

Figure 1 shows the basic structure of an immunoglobulin molecule which consists of two identical heavy and two identical light polypeptide chains that are held together by disulfide bonds. The heavy chains are antigenically distinct for each of the five classes of immunoglobulin while two types of light chains are found in all five immunoglobulin classes. However, each individual immunoglobulin molecule within a class contains only one type of light chain, either kappa or lambda. Approximately two thirds of the immunoglobulin molecules in each class possess kappa light chains and one third possess lambda.[12]

Light and heavy chains of the antibody molecule are composed of a variable and constant region. The amino acid sequence comprising the C-terminal half of the chains are identical while the N-terminal half discloses many variations. For example, the C-terminal half of the heavy chains of the IgG molecule are the same for all molecules of that class. In contrast, the N-terminal halves of the chains show considerable variaton. The variable portion of light and heavy chains is responsible for antigen recognition and is the binding site for antigen. A light chain consists of approximately 214 amino acids and a heavy chain of about twice as many. Approximately 107 of the positions constitute the variable region in light and heavy chains.

The immunoglobulin molecule can be split by proteolytic enzymes into biologically active fragments. Digestion by papain splits the molecule into three parts: two identical Fab or antigen binding fragments and one Fc fragment. Each Fab fragment consists of one complete light chain plus the amino terminal half of a heavy chain. The Fc fragment contains most of the determinants responsible for class specificity. This fragment does not combine with antigen but is the region which fixes complement, binds IgE to mast cells in immediate hypersensitivity reactions, and is responsible for antibody–dependent cellular cytotoxicity in neoplasia.

Pepsin, on the other hand, cleaves to the right of the heavy chain disulfide bonds resulting in a larger Fab fragment than papain. The Fc fragment is broken into several small pieces and is not recovered by this method.

The primary function of the antibody molecule is to selectively bind antigen. As mentioned previously, this function is localized in the Fab fragment and more specifically to the variable region. The amino acid sequence and spatial arrangement determine antigen specificity of the immunoglobulin. In general, however, it is the chemical structure of the antigen that actually determines the resulting specificity and affinity of the antibody molecule.

Another important feature in antigen-antibody reactions is avidity, i.e., the tendency of antibody to combine and form stable complexes with the antigen. Combination of antigen and antibody is specific and reversible. Therefore, there is continual dissociation of antigen and antibody in immune reactions. IgM antibodies have been shown to have at least five binding sites per molecule. These pentavalent antibodies would be expected to form less dissociable complexes with multivalent antigen than would a mono–or bivalent antobody. Thus, if the affinity for each binding site of these antibodies was similar, the pentavalent form would be more avid then either of the other two molecules.

The configuration of IgG, IgE, and IgD are simple monomers while IgA can be a monomer, dimer, or even a trimer.[13] The IgA monomers are connected by a polypeptide chain known as a J chain to form the dimer and trimer.[14] The dimer of IgA is unique

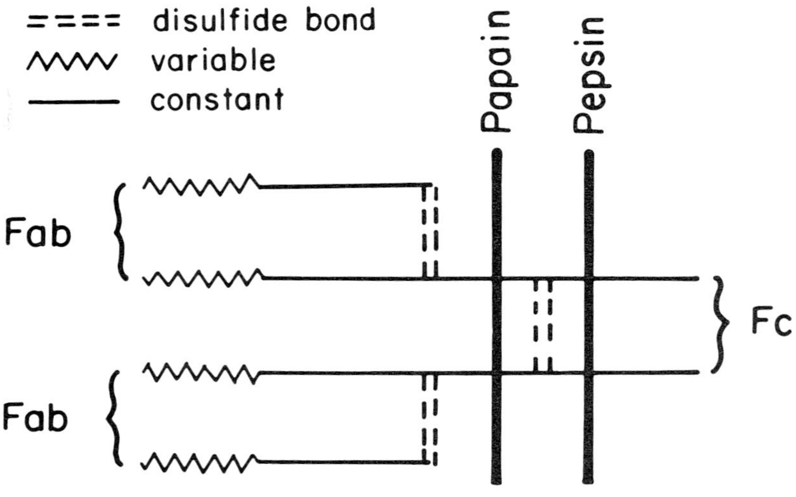

FIGURE 1. Structure of immunoglobulin molecule (IgG) illustrating cleavage by papain and pepsin.

in that a secretory nonimmunoglobulin component is firmly attached to heavy chains, probably by disulfide bonds, between the two connected monomers. This component is thought to be produced in epithelial cells rather than in immunoglobulin-producing plasma cells. The usual form of the large IgM antibody is visualized as a pentamer; i.e., five subunits joined by J chains forming a stellar configuration. Therefore, one IgM antibody actually has ten antigen combining sites, but is considered to have a valence of five since five of the sites are very weak.

III. RECOGNITION OF ANTIGEN AND CELL DIFFERENTIATION

B lymphocytes, the precursors of antibody-forming cells, possess immunoglobulins on their surface which function as receptors for antigenic determinants. Clonal selection, the accepted theory describing lymphocyte differentiation, contends that antigen selects a relatively few lymphoid cells which possess receptors for that particular antigen and subsequently these few cells proliferate and differentiate giving rise to expanded populations of antigen specific cells.[15] In other words, contact of B lymphocytes with antigen triggers clonal proliferation of a predetermined number of B cells, each of which proliferate and form a clone secreting antibody of characteristic idiotype.

There are essentially three stages of the humoral immune response: (1) triggering of B lymphocytes by antigen followed by, (2) proliferation and, finally, (3) maturation and differentiation which produce plasma cells that synthesize and release antibody as well as memory B lymphocytes (Figure 2). The antibody response to many antigens requires cooperation between B and T cells and often macrophages. The association of these cells will be discussed in Section V, "Regulation of Antibody Production."

During progression of lymphocyte differentiation, IgM is the first immunoglobulin to appear on the surface of B lymphocytes.[16] IgD is later aquired on the IgM–bearing cells. Consequently, IgM and IgD are the predominant surface isotypes of B lymphocytes. Stem cells in bone marrow acquire IgM and migrate to the spleen where they further differentiate into IgM blasts and then into small lymphocytes which bear both IgM and IgD. The IgM–bearing cells after antigen stimulation can differentiate into IgG bearing

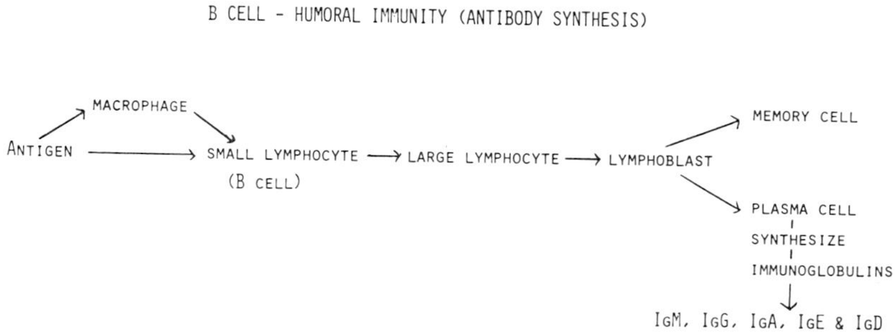

FIGURE 2. Simplified B lymphocyte pathway of humoral immunity.

cells which carry immunologic memory. IgE–producing cells, like those of the other immunoglobulin classes, arise from IgM–bearing precursor cells.[17]

Polyclonal B cell activators (PBA) should be mentioned at this point. PBA are substances which directly activate immunoglobulin cells to proliferate and secrete antibody by interacting with receptors which are not immunoglobulin receptors.[18] The activation is not immunologically specific since the variable portion of the immunoglobulin receptors is not involved. This indicates that some B cells can be activated in the absence of antigen stimulation to secrete nonspecific antibody.

IV. PRODUCTION AND SECRETION OF ANTIBODY

Introduction of antigen into a host results in either direct stimulation of B cells or the antigen may initially be phagocytized by macrophages which transfers the antigenic determinants to B lymphocytes. The sensitized small lymphocytes progress through a series of transformations into large lymphocytes and finally lymphoblasts which differentiate into antibody secreting plasma cells or small memory lymphocytes (Figure 2).

The reaction commences when antigen molecules encounter small lymphocytes with surface antibody to that particular antigen. The antigen is bound to the antibody which provokes the small lymphocytes to divide and differentiate. During differentiation, the surface antigen-antibody complexes are lost and replaced by new antibody receptors. The memory cells possess surface immunoglobulin receptors similar to the original small lymphocytes while plasma cells synthesize and secrete circulating antibody.

Each antibody producing cell makes only one type of immunoglobulin, i.e., one type of heavy chain and one type of light chain. These antibodies migrate through the circulatory and lymphatic systems combining with designated antigen and contribute to rapid elimination of the antigen from the body. Antigen can be destroyed in a variety of ways. Complement fixation may occur in some bacterial infections by provoking lysis of the cell membrane. Other antigens stimulate production of antibodies which enhance phagocytosis (opsonization). Another method is neutralization by antibody, (or antitoxin) directed against a toxin. Once the toxin is controlled, the cells producing the toxin can be destroyed by phagocytosis.

The memory cell, on the other hand, is a resting antigen sensitized B cell which responds to a second exposure to that antigen by rapid production of large amounts of antibody. These antibodies usually have a greater affinity and specificity for antigen than those produced after initial exposure.

The primary immune response represents the individual's first contact with that particular antigen. A lag phase when antibody cannot be detected is usually present for two days (Figure 3). This period is followed by an exponential rise in antibody which reaches

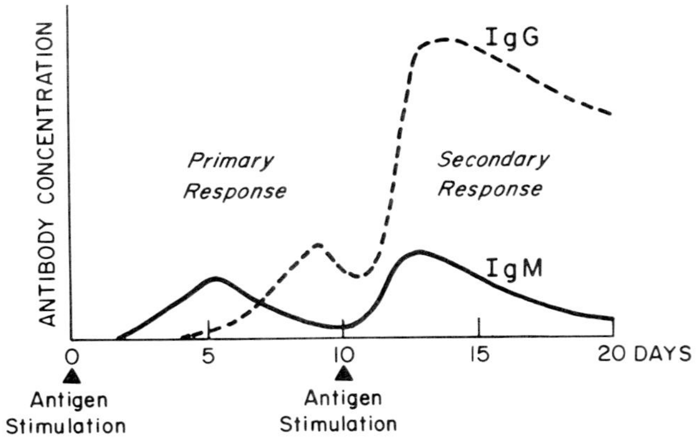

FIGURE 3. Primary and secondary immune response of IgM and IgG.

peak titer in two or three days. A phase of decline subsequently follows. IgM appears early and is the principal antibody of the primary response but later shifts to IgG.

The secondary immune response (anamnestic response) represents reexposure to the same antigen weeks, months, or even years after the primary antibody response has subsided. The secondary response has a very brief lag phase, requires lesser quantity of antigen to form the amount of antibody produced in the primary response, synthesizes antibody at an increased rate, and has a greater peak titer. The antibody which is produced (primarily IgG) persists, has a prolonged steady state, and has a greater affinity for antigen than those produced during the primary response. As mentioned previously, the secondary immune response is attributed to persistence of a substantial number of antigen-sensitive memory cells after initial contact with the antigen. IgG production is by far greater in the secondary response than primary response while IgM is similar for both responses.

IgM molecules are the first antibodies synthesized in response to antigenic stimulation. They are stimulated particularly by viruses, have a half-life in serum of approximately 5 days, fix complement well in the presence of antigen, and are synthesized in utero in the human fetus but do not cross the placental barrier. About 7% of immunoglobulin in normal serum is IgM.

IgG, on the other hand, occurs later in the immune response, has a half-life of about 23 days, can cross the human placenta and comprises more than 80% of the total serum immunoglobulins. IgG is the immunoglobulin responsible for long lasting protection to infectious agents.

IgA is the immunoglobulin of external secretions such as colostrum, saliva, tears, and secretions of the gastrointestinal, respiratory, and urogenital tracts. The IgA molecule is formed locally in plasma cells of the submucosa while the secretory component is formed in the epithelial cells. Secretory IgA is produced more effectively by local than systemic infections and antigen stimulation. IgA does not fix complement but may activate C3 by alternate pathways. Secretory IgA is active against viruses and bacteria. IgA comprises approximately 15% of the immunoglobulin in human serum.

IgE is present in minute concentration in normal serum. IgE has an important function in immediate hypersensitivity (allergic) reactions. This immunoglobulin is produced by plasma cells in mucous membranes and regional lymph nodes of the respiratory and gastrointestinal tract. After combining with antigen, the Fc region of the IgE molecule attaches to basophils and tissue mast cells. The ensuing reaction results in degranulation of these cells and the release of mediators (histamine, slow reacting substance, etc.) which cause tissue reaction (contraction of smooth muscle, secretion of exocrine glands, etc.). Individuals with allergic hypersensitivities may have a marked increase in concentrations of serum IgE.

IgD–bearing lymphocytes are found in higher concentrations in umbilical cord blood than adult blood suggesting that this immunoglobulin is a primitive recognition unit or for regulation of the immune response.[19] As many as 20% of circulating B lymphocytes may bear surface IgD which is frequently associated with IgM on the same cell.[16] Even though IgD is a prominent surface–bound immunoglobulin in the newborn, IgD is absent in the serum or may constitute only 0.2% of serum immunoglobulins.[20]

V. REGULATION OF ANTIBODY PRODUCTION

Antibody responses to many antigens require cooperation between at least two types of lymphocytes for optimal expression. Differentiation of bone marrow–derived B cells into antibody–secreting plasma cells is usually regulated by thymus–derived T cells. The function of the T cell and its soluble factor is not to produce antibody, but rather to aid in activation and proliferation of B cells.[21] A third cell type, the macrophage, also has an important role as an accessory cell by cooperating with T cells and aiding the response of B cells to antigens.

There are at least four types of T cells recognized to date. These include cytotoxic, helper, amplifier, and suppressor T cells. All but the cytotoxic lymphocyte function in regulating the humoral immune response. The helper T cell is required for activation of B cells to many antigens while the amplifier T cell regulates proliferation of activated B lymphocytes. This cooperation may occur either by cell to cell contact or by release of soluble factors by T cells.[22] The other T cell, suppressor T, is responsible for suppressing antibody synthesis by inhibiting B lymphocytes. In general, B cell activity is regulated by a balance of helper and suppressor T cells. Exposure to a weak or small antigen dose may induce helper T cells while a strong antigen or larger dose may induce suppressor T cells thereby controlling amount of antibody synthesized.

The helper T cell, as described previously, is required for initiation and actually triggers B cells for antibody synthesis. This function can occur by direct contact of T and B cells or by release of soluble factors from activated T lymphocytes. T cells are known to be able to assist in producing IgM, IgG, IgA, and IgE. This cooperation appears to be restricted in that a single T cell activates a single B cell precursor [23] but an increase in helper cell numbers may result in a disproportionately larger increase in amount of antibody produced.[21] Helper T cells also seem to convey their greatest effect on B cells at lower dosages of antigen.[24]

The amplifier T lymphocyte tends to regulate rather than initiate antibody formation. The purpose of this cell is to increase the magnitude of the antibody response.[25]

Suppressor T cells, on the other hand, suppress antibody synthesis by B lymphocytes. Suppressor T activity can be identified in mice before B cell function matures and, therefore, is thought to contribute to unresponsiveness generated by self and other antigens during the neonatal period as well as prevention of autoimmune disease.[25] Suppressor T cells are also present in large quantities in old mice and are considered to be responsible for age-related immunosuppression.[26]

Suppressor T cells limit B cell proliferation in response to antigen by limiting clone size. The suppressor T cell is directed primarily towards B cell precursors by halting proliferation or preventing their differentiation into antibody–forming cells. They have been known to interfere with production of IgM, IgG, and IgE. Suppressor T cells also interfere with helper and amplifier T cells.[25]

The IgG response is considerably more dependent on the helper T cell than is the IgM response.[27,28] T cells are not necessary for induction of memory in B cells but T cells or soluble factors derived from activated T cells are important in expression of B memory upon challenge.[29] Furthermore, a greater antibody response can occur if the number of antigen-activated T cells increases independently of B cells.[15] These T cells recirculate long after exposure to antigen and are thought to account in part for memory.

Macrophages are also modulators of humoral immunity. Macrophages, like B lymphocytes, have receptors for complement and the Fc portion of immunoglobulin. One function of macrophages is to localize antigen and bring it closer to an antibody-forming lymphocyte. Macrophages may also process antigen in lysosomes making it highly antigenic.[30,31,32] It is not exactly clear how the macrophage-antigen interaction results in enhanced antigen immunogenicity but it is known that both antigen-induced lymphocyte proliferation and the differentiation of antibody-forming cells from lymphocyte precursors during the primary response in vitro require the assistance of macrophages.[33] Like the T-B cell interaction, this cooperation may occur by physical contact between the macrophage and B cell or by soluble factors released from the macrophage. Macrophages also activate T lymphocytes to produce nonspecific helper activity for antibody production.[34,35]

In summary, the pathway of the humoral immune system from antigen stimulation to antibody synthesis is extremely complex. The B lymphocyte is the progenitor of antibody-forming plasma cells but optimum responses are not usually achieved without participation by T lymphocytes and macrophages. Furthermore, it is a balance between helper T and suppressor T as well as amplifier T and macrophages that regulate B cell activity and consequently the humoral immune response.

VI. COMPLEMENT

Complement consists of 11 proteins present in the blood of all vertebrates including man. These proteins act to amplify and enhance the efficiency of the humoral immune system. Proteins of the complement system respond to the complex between antibody and antigen (classically a cell membrane antigen) by combining with receptors on the Fc portion of the antibody molecule and, via a series of enzymatic activation steps, lead to damage or lysis of the foreign cell membrane. Further effects of this immune reaction result in the tissue changes associated with inflammation and subsequent containment of pathogens within the site.

The 11 proteins of the complement system comprise about 10% of serum globulins mostly of the beta (β) class (Table 1). These glycoproteins are not immunoglobulins, are not increased by immunization, nor are they specific for antigen or antibody. The complement reaction is heat labile (mostly the C1 component), Mg^{++} and Ca^{++} dependent, and fixes only to antibody complexed with multivalent antigen. It is thought that the steric alteration of antibody complexed with antigen reveals the complement binding site on the Fc fragment. Immunoglobulins vary in their capacity to bind complement. Complement is bound readily by IgM and to a lesser extent by IgG (IgG_1, IgG_2, IgG_3 subclasses in order of effectiveness).

The complement proteins are designated in numerical order of their role in the reaction except for C4 (appears before C2) which was named before identification of the actual sequence was described. A bar (i.e., $C\overline{4,2}$) over the numbers is used to specify an activated or enzyme form. Enzymatic-cleavage fragments of complement components are designated with lower case letters such as C3a or C3b.

Table 1
PROPERTIES OF HUMAN COMPLEMENT COMPONENTS

Component	Serum conc. μg/mℓ	S-Rate[a]	Mol wt	Electrophoretic mobility
Cl	—	19.0	600,000	—
Clq	180	11.1	400,000	γ2
Clr	—	7.5	180,000	β
Cls	110	4.5	86,000	α
C2	25	4.5	117,000	β1
C3	1600	9.5	180,000	β2
C3a	—	—	8,900	—
C4	640	10.0	206,000	β1
C5	80	8.7	180,000	β1
C5a	—	—	16,500	—
C6	75	5.5	95,000	β2
C7	55	6.0	110,000	β2
C8	80	8.0	163,000	γ1
C9	230	4.5	79,000	α

[a] Sedimentation coefficient (S).

Discussion of the series of reactions that follow initiation of the complement system can best be discerned if divided into three stages: recognition, activation, and membrane attack. A pictorial representation of Muller-Eberhard's[36] three site model of the complement system is presented in Figure 4. The steps of this model are described below.

RECOGNITION — The first (Cl) component of complement is comprised of three proteins (Clq, Clr, Cls). The Clq protein combines with the Fc receptor on the antibody molecule (IgM or IgG) complexed with antigen and undergoes conformational change activating the proenzyme Clr, which in turn converts Cls to the active $\overline{\text{Cls}}$ (serine protease).

ACTIVATION — The $\overline{\text{Cls}}$ moiety is instrumental in furthering events in the classical complement pathway acting on C4 by cleaving it into two fragments, C4a and C4b. The C4b fragment has a short-lived active site which enables it to combine with a membrane receptor. Only those C4b fragments that quickly become membrane-bound participate in further reactions. All others become inactive and remain in the blood stream. In the next step, $\overline{\text{Cls}}$ cleaves C2 into C2a and C2b. The C2a component binds with membrane–bound C4b resulting in active C3 convertase $\overline{\text{C4b,2a}}$. The $\overline{\text{C4,2}}$ component then cleaves C3 into C3a and C3b at which time C3b becomes associated with $\overline{\text{C4,2}}$ creating $\overline{\text{C4,2,3}}$ or C5 convertase. The smaller fragment C3a known as anaphylatoxin has potent biologic properties which along with C5a augment the inflammatory reaction.

MEMBRANE ATTACK — The C5 convertase $\overline{\text{C4,2,3}}$ next cleaves C5 into C5a and C5b fragments. As mentioned above, C5a has anaphylatoxin activity whereas C5b continues to further the complement reaction. At this point, the self-assembling process is initiated and no further enzyme activity occurs. Subsequently, C5b,6,7 are assembled together providing a binding region for C8. The C,5,6,7,8 complex further furnishes a binding region for six C9 proteins. The C5-9 complex is able to attach to membrane determinants by the C5 moiety and cause membrane damage and/or cell lysis. The specifics fo cell damage or lysis are unclear, however, after C8 and C9 are bound, minute "holes" appear (as seen by electron microscopy) in the membrane. These membrane lesions and the resultant loss of membrane integrity lead to lysis or permanent cell damage.

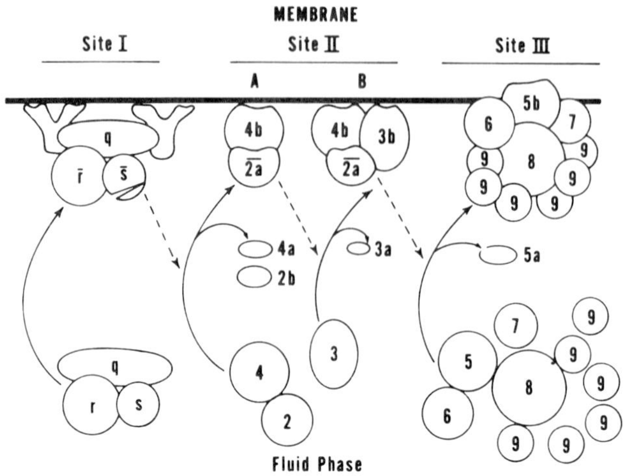

FIGURE 4. A pictorial representation of Muller-Eberhard's[36] three site model of the complement system is presented. The recognition step occurs at Site I between C1 and membrane-bound antibody. Activation involves enzymatic reactions at Site II between $C\overline{1s}$, C4, C2, and C3. The final membrane attack sequence occurs at Site III with the remaining components, C5,6,7,8,9. Details of the classical complement system are described in the text.

In addition to the classic complement pathway there exists an alternate or properdin pathway that does not require antigen-antibody complexes to activate the reaction. The alternate pathway commences with activation of C3 and proceeds with the assembly of the other complement constituents as with the classical pathway.

The alternate complement pathway can be activated by agents such as endotoxin (lipopolysaccharide from cell walls of Gram–negative bacteria), zymosan (polysaccharide from yeast cell walls), and aggregated antibodies such as IgA and IgE.[2] Much attention has been focused in recent years to the events that follow activation prior to cleavage of C3. Studies are underway to identify the enzymes and reactions equivalent to the first steps seen with the classical pathway.[36]

The alternate pathway is less efficient at bringing about membrane damage and cell lysis than the classic pathway, however, it may play an important roll in augmentation of an inflammatory response (via C3a and C5a) especially when specific antibody is in low concentration.

The complement reaction can have potent effects on cells and tissues. The generation of anaphylatoxin fragments C3a and C5a effect the release of histamine from mast cells mediating an increase in capillary permeability, contraction of smooth muscle, as well as chemotactic migration of polymorphonuclear leukocytes. Cell–bound C3b and C5b are responsible for immune adherance and opsonization which is probably instrumental in phagocytosis. The final sequence of events in the classical complement pathway lead to cell membrane damage and in some cases cytolysis.

The activities generated by complement are, in cost cases, beneficial due mostly to the specificity of the reaction and built-in control mechanisms. Control is imparted via several serum inhibitors such as a C1s inhibitor that destroys C1, a C3b inactivator that destroys $C\overline{4,2,3}$ as well as immune adherance properties, and an anaphylatoxin (C3a and C5a) inactivator carboxypeptidase B.[36] Further control is evident over the C5b-9 complex due to the transient binding capacity of the complex onto the cell membrane. The C4b fragment also has a short–lived active site for the appropriate membrane receptor.

In conclusion, the primary function of complement is to enhance the action of antibody by bringing about cell membrane damage, cytolysis in some cases, and participating in inflammatory responses. The classical complement system is comprised of 11 distinct serum proteins that require antigen-antibody complexes to initiate the 3 step reaction sequence of recognition, enzymatic activation, and membrane attack. An alternate pathway is antigen-antibody independent and commences with activation of C3 by polysacchrides and certain aggregated immunoglobulins. This alternative system probably plays more of a role in inflammation than in direct cell damage or destruction. Thus, important features of the complement system lie in amplification of the humoral immune response and the destruction of pathogens.

REFERENCES

1. **Greaves, M. F., Owen, J. J. T., and Raff, M. C.,** *T and B Lymphocytes,* American Elsevier, New York, 1974.
2. **Eisen, H. N.,** *Immunology,* Harper and Row Publishers, Hagerstown, Md, 1974, 460 and 512.
3. **Owen, J. J. T., Cooper, M. D., and Raff, M. C.,** In vitro generation of B lymphocytes in mouse foetal liver, a mammalian 'bursa equivalent', *Nature (London)* 249 361, 1974.
4. **Mitchell, G. F. and Miller, J. F. A. P.,** Cell to cell interaction in the immune response. II. The source of hemolysin-forming cells in irradiated mice given bone marrow and thymus or thoracic duct lymphocytes, *J. Exp. Med.,* 128, 821, 1968.
5. **Melchers, F., Von Boehmer, H., and Phillips, R. A.,** B Lymphocyte subpopulations in the mouse, *Transplant. Rev.,* 25, 27, 1975.
6. **Nossal, G. J. V. and Schrader, J. W.,** B Lymphocyte-Antigen interactions in the initiation of tolerance or immunity, *Transplant. Rev.,* 23, 138, 1975.
7. **Osmond, D. G.,** Formation and maturation of bone marrow lymphocytes. *J. Reticuloendothelial Soc.,* 17, 99, 1975.
8. **Buckley, R. H.,** The functions and measurement of human B and T lymphocytes, *J. Invest. Dermatol.,* 67, 381, 1976.
9. **Nussenzweig, V.,** *Adv. Immunol.,* 19, 217, 1974.
10. **Bianco, C., Patrick, R., and Nussenweig, V.,** A population of lymphocytes bearing a membrane receptor or antigen-antibody complement complexes, *J. Exp. Med.,* 132, 702, 1970.
11. **Ryan, J. L. and Henkort, P. A.,** Inhibition of B lymphocyte activation by interaction with Fc receptors, *Immunol. Commun.,* 5, 455, 1976.
12. **Maddison, S. E.,** Structure and function of human immunoglobulins, *Health Lab. Sci.,* 9, 167, 1972.
13. **Good, R. A. and Fisher, D. W.,** *Immunobiology,* Sinauer Assoc., Inc., Stamford, Conn., 1971, pp. 79.
14. **Mestecky, J., Zikan, J., and Butler, W. T.,** Immunoglobulin M and secretory immunoglobulin A: presence of a common polypeptide chain different from light chains, *Science,* 171, 1163, 1971.
15. **Rowley, D. A., Fitch, F. W., Stuart, F. P., Kohler, H., and Cosenza, H.,** Specific suppression of immune responses, *Science,* 181, 1133, 1973.
16. **Vitetta, E. S., Cambier, J., Forman, J., Keltman, J. R., Yuan, D., and Uhr, J. W.,** Immunoglobulin Receptors on Marine B Lymphocytes, *Cold Spring Harbor Symp. Quantit. Biol.,* 41, 185, 1977.
17. **Mannning, D. D., Manning, J. K., and Reed, H. D.,** Suppression of reaginic antibody (IgE) formation in mice by treatment with Anti-μ Antiserum, *J. Exp. Med.,* 144, 288, 1976.
18. **Primi, D., Hammarstrom, L., Smith, C. I. E., and Moller, G.,** Characterization of self-reactive B cells by polyclonal B-cell activators, *J. Exp. Med.,* 145, 21, 1977.
19. **Abney, E. R. and Parkhouse, R. M. E.,** Candidate for Immunoglobulin D Present on Marine B lymphocytes, *Nature (London),* 252, 600, 1974.
20. **Van Boxel, J. A.,** IgD on cell membranes of human lymphoid cell lines with multiple immunoglobulin classes, *Nature (London),* 251, 443, 1974.
21. **Janeway, C. A.,** Cellular cooperation during in vivo anti-hapten antibody responses. I. the effect of cell number on the response, *J. Immunol.,* 114, 1394, 1975.
22. **Yu, H. and Gordon, J.,** Helper function in antibody synthesis mediated by soluble factors, *Nature (London) New Biol.,* 244, 20, 1973.

23. **Waldman, H., Lefkovits, I., and Feinstein, A.,** Restriction in the functions of single helper T cells, *Immunology,* 31, 353, 1976.
24. **Birnbaum, G., Weksler, M. E., and Siskind, G. W.,** Cross-reactivity of T cell helper function, *Clin. Exp. Immunol.,* 17, 55, 1974.
25. **Baker, P. J.,** Homeostatic control of antibody responses: a model based on the recognition of cell-associated antibody by regulatory T cells, *Transplant. Rev.,* 26, 3, 1975.
26. **Segre, D. and Segre, M.,** Humoral immunity in aged mice. II. Increased suppressor T cell activity in immunologically deficient old mice, *J. Immunol.,* 116, 735, 1976.
27. **Anderson, H. R., Dresser, D. W., and Wortis, H. H.,** The relationship between the immunoglobulin class of B-Cell precursors and the degree of synergism obtained from the presence of T cells, *Clin. Exp. Immunol.,* 16, 393, 1974.
28. **Paraskeras, F. and Lee, S. T.,** The helper cell function of primed T Cells, *Eur. J. Immunol.,* 6, 856, 1976.
29. **Schrader, J. W.,** The role of T Cells in IgG production; thymus-dependent antigens induce B cell memory in the absence of T Cells, *J. Immunol.,* 114, 1665, 1975.
30. **Nakano, K. and Muramatsu, S.,** Studies on the role of macrophages in the antibody response of mice: stimulation of T cell-dependent antibody responses by tolerogenic soluble antigen trapped by macrophages, *J. Reticuloendothelial Soc.,* 19, 347, 1976.
31. **Walker, W. S.,** Functional heterogenicity of macrophages in the induction and expression of acquired immunity, *J. Reticuloendothelial Soc.,* 20, 57, 1976.
32. **Lipscomb, M. F., Ben-Sasson, S. Z., and Uhr, J. W.,** Specific binding of T lymphocytes to macrophages. I. kinetics of binding, *J. Immunol.,* 118, 1748, 1977.
33. **Nielsen, M. H., Jensen, H., Braendstrup, O., and Werdelin, Q.,** Macrophage-lymphocyte clusters in the immune response to soluble protein antigen in vitro, *J. Exp. Med.,* 140, 1260, 1974.
34. **Erb, P. and Feldman, M.,** The role of macrophages in the generation of T helper cells, *Eur. J. Immunol.,* 5, 759, 1975.
35. **Jackway, J. P., Thomas, D. W., and Talmage, D. W.,** Activation of T lymphocyte helper function by brief exposure to antigen-pulsed macrophages, *Proc. Soc. Exp. Biol. Med.,* 150, 791, 1975.
36. **Muller-Eberhard, H. S.,** Complement *Ann. Rev. Biochem.,* 44, 697, 1975.

Chapter 4

CELLULAR IMMUNITY

R. P. Sharma

TABLE OF CONTENTS

I. ORIGIN AND DIFFERENTIATION OF T LYMPHOCYTES

Similar to other immunocytes, the T lymphocytes are derived from stem cells produced in the bone marrow. The migration of lymphocytes to thymus for further differentiation occurs early in life, since thymus is partially involuted with advanced age, and thymectomy at a later time in age has little influence on the immune competence. After the stem cells are accumulated in thymus they may differentiate and localize in the thymic cortex area. These cells undergo a constant multiplication and only a small portion of them is actually released from this organ. A majority of these cells actually disintegrate in the thymus itself. The cells that leave the thymus do not normally return to this organ but are localized in the secondary lymphoid organs, principally in defined areas called thymus-dependent zones.

Thymus-dependent lymphocytes or T cells are recognized by the presence of thy antigens as well as other histocompatibility antigens present on their surface. The membrane surface of T cells is believed to be devoid of immunoglobulins. Using surface markers for thymus antigens it has been demonstrated that 90% of the lymphocytes in the thymus possess these on their membranes. In the mouse nearly 65% of the lymphocytes in spleen and 85% in lymph nodes and peripheral blood are T cells. Rarely are any T cells present in the bone marrow.[1] In humans, 60-75% of the cells in blood, spleen, or lymph nodes have been characterized as T cells.[2] Human T lymphocytes possess, and are often characterized by the presence of, receptors for sheep erythrocytes and form rosettes with these cells. Rabbit peripheral blood lymphocytes are primarily T cells that may have immunoglobulins on their membranes.[3] T cells are believed to be relatively less sensitive to x-irradiation and suppression by corticosteroids as compared to the B cells but are rapidly inactivated by antilymphocytic serum.[4] T lymphocytes respond to various phytomitogens. For example, soluble concanavalin A (Con A) possesses a selective mitogenic property to immature T cells, while the mature T cells respond to phytohemagglutinin (PHA).

II. T LYMPHOCYTE SUBPOPULATIONS

Several subpopulations of T cells have been characterized. T cells are important in the recognition process after an antigen has been concentrated by a macrophage. In the mouse, one subpopulation of T cells is relatively rich in thy antigen, generally homes to the spleen, and has a short half-life.[1,4] A second subpopulation, having a lower thy concentration, generally homes to lymph nodes and has a longer half-life. It is possible that these two subpopulations represent different stages of cell maturation, the first (T_1) being evolved into the second (T_2). This maturation process may require the presence of antigen-specific stimulation.

Interactions between different types of T cells are implicated in the regulation of immune processes. The "helper" T cells usually aid maturation and clonal division of differentiated T cells, whereas another type of T cells, the "suppressor" cells, are believed to depress the function of sensitized cells. These cooperations, although convincingly demonstrated, have not been fully understood.[4]

It has been shown that T cells are required for certain B cell functions.[5] Treatment of T cells with mitomycin C impaired their "helper" activity, suggesting that T cells must be activated by the antigen to differentiate and to produce some factors that trigger B lymphocytes.[6] Recognition of the antigen by the antibody-forming cells requires two determinants; one directly by the receptor immunoglobulin molecule on B cells, and the other a "carrier" antibody secreted by T lymphocytes subsequent to the antigen recognition.[7] Antigen alone will cause immune paralysis whereas the cells are differentiated into plasma cells in the presence of a specific factor from T cells.[8]

III. T CELL RECEPTOR

In contrast to the B lymphocytes which have immunoglobulins on their surface, there is evidence to indicate that the membrane receptors on T cells are not immunoglobulins. Although the characteristics and nature of the T cell-receptor are not fully understood, it has been suggested that the receptors on these cells are β_2-microglobulin, a small component of the immunoglobulin molecule.[9] The similarity between the β_2-microglobulin and the histocompatibility antigen has been suggested. The presence of this small protein has been shown on T cell surfaces. Antibodies prepared against this microglobulin inhibit the mitogenic response of lymphocytes to specific T cell stimulants.

An IgM-like receptor has been isolated from the T lymphocyte membranes.[10] This macromolecule binds antigens and complexes with macrophages. Monomeric IgM, however, does not bind to B or T lymphocytes, and a similar fraction isolated from the B lymphocytes was unable to bind macrophages.

The exact nature of other receptors that bind mitogenic substances is not understood. It has been shown that both T and B cells will bind different lectins that are selective mitogens for the two types of lymphocytes, whereas only one subpopulation of the cells may show a mitogenic effect.[11]

IV. LYMPHOKINES

A number of soluble factors are produced by T lymphocytes and these biologically active substances are called lymphokines.[12,13] Possibly other types of lymphoid cells other than T cells may be involved in the production of lymphokines. Although many of these have not been characterized and possibly involve several components, a number of them are proteins or glycoproteins. A majority of these are heat-stable and are effectively degraded by chymotrypsin.

A list of selected lymphokines that have been described is given in Table 1. The lymphokines are often classified according to the nature of the effector cells on which they act (e.g., macrophage migration inhibition factor) or by the type of activity (i.e., cytotoxic or chemotactic factors). It is not clear whether the cells that release lymphokines are the same that proceed to clonal proliferation. The exact mechanism in which these factors are produced by the cells is not well characterized.

The lymphokines have their effects on macrophages, other lymphocytes or even other types of tissue cells. Interferon, a substance secreted by T cells protects the cells from viral antigens. Other factors cause aggregation of cells, inhibit their migration, activate or suppress the mitotic division in cells or may cause lytic or cytotoxic action on effector cells. The list of lymphokines is likely to be increased as more factors are brought to light and the molecular mechanisms of immune reactions are further investigated. It is likely that some of the factors listed in Table 1 are identical and have different types of effects on different cells.

V. MACROPHAGES AND IMMUNITY

The role of macrophages and the cells in reticuloendothelial system in immune responsiveness has been well established. The macrophages are relatively less sensitive to radiation damage but the phagocytic activity of these cells may be different from their role in the modulation of immune responses.[14] For example, the macrophages exposed

Table 1
VARIOUS LYMPHOKINES PRODUCED BY LYMPHOCYTES

Factors	Function	Abbreviation
Chemotactic factors	Aggregation of macrophage	CFM
	Aggregation of lymphocytes	CFL
	Aggregation of PMN leukocytes	CFP
Migration inhibition factors for macrophage	Antigen-independent inhibition	MIF
	Antigen–specific inhibition	SMIF
Mitogenic factors	Lymphocyte transformation	MF or LTF
	Antigen-dependent B cell mitosis or nonspecific factor	LMF or NSF
Macrophage stimulating factors	Activation of macrophage	MAF
	Specific factor	SMAF
Lymphocyte maturation factors	Specific (Thymus replacing)	IgT
	Nonspecific for B cell maturation	NSF
Lymphotoxin	Cytostatic	LT
Proliferation inhibitory	Prevents transformation	PIF
Skin reactive ractor	Causes skin reaction	SRF
Interferon	Protects cells from viruses	IF
Transfer factor	Transfer of immunity	TF
Complement inhibitor	Prevents complement-dependent cytotoxicity	CI

to radiation will accumulate the injected particulate material whereas other immunologic effects, such as antigen processing within these cells, are greatly impaired. The role of the macrophage in immune reactions depends on the type of antigen. There is no agreement whether the RNA-complexing of antigen in the macrophages is a necessary step for the development of immunity against antigens that involve participation of these cells. It has been suggested that the antigen on the surface of these cells, rather than the one contained within, is responsible for the immunological potential of macrophage-associated antigens.[15] It is likely that the arrangement of antigenic material on the macrophage surface somehow can be important for the antigen recognition by other lymphoid cells. A lattice of antigenic determinants may be formed on the macrophage surface and the immunocompetent cells may be stimulated when they encounter the antigen having repeating units.

The macrophages are also important in bringing different types of cells close to each other so that cell cooperativity may occur. Cell clusters formed around the adherent cells have been shown to be necessary for an optimal production of antibodies in vitro.[16]

It is possible that viable macrophages are needed to achieve immunological maturity. This has been indicated because neonatal rabbits lack immunocompetence and the injection of peritoneal macrophages results in the enhancement of immunological reactivity against an antigen.[17] The immunological function was not restored if nonviable macrophages were administered. Similarly, neonatal mice also lack immunocompetent lymphoid cells,[18] and are perhaps deficient in the immunologic recognition system that involves macrophages. Macrophages exert an important control over the rate of DNA synthesis and cell proliferation of lymphoid cells.

Supernatants from the peritoneal cells appear to reverse the depression of immunity in an in vitro system caused by the removal of macrophages.[19] This suggested that the macrophages may secrete humoral substances that stimulate the immune reactivity. In other experiments the presence of intact macrophages has been shown to cause suppression of immune responses. It appears that the macrophages are not needed in every immune response, but selective types of immune mechanisms may either be potentiated or suppressed by the presence of these cells.

The activity of macrophages may be controlled by the soluble substances that are released by the T lymphocytes. Some of these factors have been indicated earlier in this chapter. These include migration inhibition factor, chemotactic factor, pinocytosis activating factor, and specific or nonspecific macrophage activating factors.

VI. GENERAL MECHANISMS INVOLVED IN CELL-MEDIATED IMMUNITY

The exact molecular mechanisms that are involved in the cell mediated immunity are still far from clear. Cell-mediated immunity differs from the humoral immune mechanisms since the latter involves direct neutralization of the antigenic substance by preformed molecules (antibodies). In the case of cell-mediated immunity the effects require a close proximity or a direct contact between the affector lymphoid cells and the target tissue cells. The reaction is usually localized in contrast to the generalized phenomenon possible in humoral immune mechanisms.

Based on various findings of in vivo and in vitro experimentation to characterize the cell-mediated immunity, a general scheme of events can be constructed.[12] The overall sequence can be considered as (1) specific antigen recognition, (2) an amplification phase, and (3) expression of response. The first phase involves an activation of a small number of reactive lymphocytes. This activation may result in the production of various lymphhokines, such as chemotactic factors that will attract other lymphocytes or monocytes to the site. The insensitized lymphocytes can be activated by various mitogenic factors, and hence amplification of response may occur. This process can be repeated for further amplification. The infiltrated monocytes are activated to macrophages by specific macrophage arming factors (SMAF). These activated cells show increased phagocytic activity and increased lysosomal action. The activated cells, including lymphocytes and macrophages, can now cause cytotoxic reactions by subsequent release of biologically active molecules or by phagocytic mechanisms.

A classic example of cell-mediated immunity is illustrated by the one involved in an allograft rejection. No antibodies are involved in this phenomenon and neither B lymphocytes nor macrophages are required. The reaction is specific since the presence of a different transplantation antigen is not influenced. The process is a delayed one, requiring a week or more. In the case of tumor-antigen–induced cytotoxicity, the macrophages play an important role and the process involves a rather nonspecific killing of target cells. In case of K-cell-mediated cytotoxicity, the antibodies fixed on tissue surfaces initiate a specific response that can involve macrophages and also nonphagocytic K cells, that are believed to be specially differentiated T cells.

REFERENCES

1. **Raff, M. C. and Cantor, H.,** Subpopulations of thymus cells and thymus derived cells, in *Progress in Immunology,* Amos, B., Ed., Academic Press, New York, 1971.
2. **Silveira, N. P. A., Mendes, N. F., and Tolnai, M. E. A.,** Tissue localization of two populations of human lymphocytes distinguished by membrane receptors, *J. Immunol,* 108, 1456, 1972.
3. **Sell, S. and Sheppard, H. W.,** Rabbit blood lymphocytes may be T cells with surface immunoglobulins, *Science,* 182, 586, 1973.
4. **Sell, S.,** *Immunology, Immunopathology and Immunity,* 2nd ed., Harper and Row, Hagerstown, Md., 1975.

5. **Blackstock, R., Hyde, R. M., and Maserang, D. L.,** The role of thymus and bone marrow cells in immunologic competence, *South. Med. J.*, 69, 209, 1976.
6. **Miller, J. F. A. P., Sprent, J., and Basten, A. L.,** Cell to cell interaction in the immune response. VII. Requirement for differentiation of thymus derived cells, *J. Exp. Med.*, 134, 1266, 1971.
7. **Bretscha, P. A. and Cohn, M.,** A theory of self-nonself discrimination, *Science,* 169, 1042, 1970.
8. **Feldman, M. and Basten, A.,** Cell interactions in the immune response in vitro. IV. Comparison of the effects of antigen specific and allogeneic thymus-derived cell factors, *J. Exp. Med.*, 136, 722, 1972.
9. **Bach, M. L., Huang, S. W., Hong, R., and Poulik, M. D.,** β_2-microglobulin: Association with lymphocyte receptors, *Science,* 182, 1350, 1973.
10. **Cone, R. E., Feldman, M., and Marchalonis, J. J.,** Cytophilic properties of surface immunoglobulin of thymus-derived lymphocytes, *Immunology,* 26, 49, 1974.
11. **Möller, G.,** Lymphocyte activation by mitogens, *Transplant. Rev.*, 11, 1, 1972.
12. **Valdimarsson, H.,** Effector mechanisms in cellular immunity, in *The Immune System,* Hobart, M. J. and McConnell, I. Eds., Blackwell Scientific, Oxford, 1975.
13. **Synderman, R., and Pike, M. C.,** The role of lymphokines in delayed hypersensitivity reactions, in *Immunopharmacology,* Rosenthale, M. E. and Mansmann, H. C., Eds., Spectrum Publications, New York, 1975.
14. **Blackstock, R. and Hyde, R. M.,** The role of thymus and bone marrow cells in immunlogic competence. I. *South. Med. J.*, 69, 97, 1976.
15. **Schmidtke, J. R. and Uranue, E. R.,** Macrophage-antigen interaction. Uptake, metabolism and immunogenecity of foreign albumin, *J. Immunol.*, 107, 331, 1971.
16. **Pierce, C. W.,** Immune responses in vitro. Independence of activated lymphoid cells, *J. Reticuloendothel. Soc.*, 7, 647, 1970.
17. **Martin, W. J.,** Cellular basis of immunological tolerance in newborn animals, *Aust. J. Exp. Biol. Med. Sci.*, 44, 605, 1966.
18. **Braun, W. and Lasky, L. J.,** Antibody formation in newborn mice initiated through adult macrophages, *Fed. Proc. Fed. Am. Soc. Exp. Bio.*, 26, 642, 1967.
19. **Hoffman, M.,** Peritoneal macrophages in the immune to sRBC in vitro, *Immunology* 18, 791, 1970.
20. **Bloom, B. R.,** In vitro mechanisms of cell-mediated immune reactions, *Adv. Immunol.*, 13, 102, 1971.

Chapter 5

TISSUE OR CELL INJURY IN IMMUNE MECHANISMS

R. P. Sharma

TABLE OF CONTENTS

I. INTRODUCTION

The primary purpose of the immune responses is to cause the elimination of foreign or invading materials, or cells such as bacteria, other parasites, tumors, or incompatible tissues. In many cases the mechanisms involved are also harmful to the host system. A number of cells or tissues in the host organism can be damaged by immune mechanisms and lead to variable degrees of problems. The study of harmful conditions produced as a result of immune responses is referred to as *immunopathology*. In some cases the tissues are damaged subsequent to the initial neutralization of the foreign target-molecule or cell-component. The factors released from the immunocompetent cells can cause tissue inflammation which may be ultimately advantageous to the host organism but nonetheless cytotoxic in nature.

Normal tissues are considered damaged if they are recognized as "foreign" by the immune system. Nearly any tissue can be damaged if an immunity can be acquired against it. Table 1 lists a number of conditions generally produced subsequent to the immunological responses. They have been classified as type I — IV reactions according to the mechanism involved in producing cell or tissue injury.[1] The term *allergic reactions* is sometimes used to describe the immunologically caused responses.

In antigen-antibody neutralization reactions, it is usually the endothelial lining of blood vessels that is involved in the damage reaction. Other reactions may be localized if the route of entry and subsequent distribution of an antigen is limited to a confined tissue area. Generalized reactions such as anaphylaxis involve a number of organs or systems because the effects are produced by the release of biologically active substances from the affected cells.

II. FACTORS IMPLICATED IN TISSUE INJURY

A. Lymphokines

The substances produced by lymphocytes have important effects on other immunocompetent factors of host cells. One biological function of these factors in tissues is the production of inflammation. A description of these factors has been given earlier (Chapter 4). The cytotoxic factor released by the sensitized lymphocytes upon contact with the antigen causes destruction of target cells in vitro. The factor may be nonspecific in nature and may cause lysis of any cell in the vicinity. Another one, the skin–reactive factor, is similar to the macrophage migration inhibition factor. Released by sensitized lymphocytes this factor causes an inflammatory response when produced or injected in the skin.

The accumulation and activation of lymphocytes and macrophages is perhaps necessary at the inflammatory site for defense against antigenic cells. The accumulation of immune affector cells at the site of delayed hypersensitivity is aided by the production of various lymphokines by initial action of specific and active lymphocytes. Immunologic amplification would ensue at the site of reaction when more immunocytes are recruited to produce additional active factors.

B. Enzymes and Their Activation

There is growing evidence that the activation of immunocompetent cells involves an initial effect on various cellular enzymes, including esterases and lysozymes. Secretion of histamine and serotonin by mast cells, basophils, and platelets is believed to be induced by esterase activation.[2] Processes like chemotaxis and erythrophagocytosis may also involve esterase activation. Activation of esterases is implicated in lysozomal enzyme secretions by neutrophils and the antibody-induced movement of lymphocytes.

Table 1
IMMUNOPATHOLOGIC MECHANISMS IN TISSUE INJURY

Immunologic nature	Type of responses	General mechanisms	Examples of associated problems
Humoral	I	Anaphylactic reactions: release of active substances by antigen reaction with IgE fixed on target cells	Hay fever, cutaneous or systemic anaphylaxis, penicillin allergy
Humoral	II	Fixation of antigen on a target cell, reaction with antibody resulting in complement induced cytotoxicity	Hemolytic anemia, transfusion reactions, autoallergic diseases
Humoral	III	Antigen-antibody complex precipitating on cells, reaction complement dependent	Arthus reaction, serum sickness, glomerulonephritis, Goodpastures' syndrome, amyloidosis
Cellular	IV	Delayed hypersensitivity, antigen-sensitized cells causing cytotoxic effect	Tuberculin reaction, graft rejection, tumor associated conditions
Humoral	—	Antibody production to biologically important molecules (e.g., insulin or clotting factors) or normal tissues	Allergic diabetes, hemophilia, myasthenia gravis, pernicious anemia, allergic encephalomyelitis

Becker[3] has reviewed the possible role of esterase enzymes and the evidence that these enzymes are activated in a number of immunological mechanisms. In general, the evidence that activation of an esterase is required is provided by the fact that immunological functions are inhibited by well known esterase inhibitors, i.e., organophosphorus compounds. The extent of interference of an immunological mechanism was well correlated with the esterase-inhibiting property of the compound employed.

The above author[3] suggested the possibility of employing specific organophosphates for therapeutic use as immunosuppressants. In some of the studies reviewed, a modification of the chemical structure resulted in a very specific action on immunologic functions. Because of the toxic effects of potent organophosphates, a selective chemical is not yet available. It is likely that the immunosuppressive properties of organophosphorus insecticides are mediated via their inhibition of esterase-dependent activities in the immune functions.

Other lysosomal enzymes important in the destruction of phagocytized materials by neutrophils include acid phosphatase, β-glucuronidase, cathepsin, and other acid hydrolases. Many of these are toxic to host cells.

C. Histamine

This potent biologically active substance is synthesized and stored in a number of cell types including mast cells, basophils, or platelets. The interaction of a specific antigen with cell-bound antibody, IgE, on the surface of these cells will cause the expulsion of this mediator. Release of histamine is responsible for various events in anaphylaxis and other allergic reactions. The effects of histamine include bronchoconstriction, capillary dilatation, increased capillary permeability, and increased exocrine secretions in various organs. These effects lead to hypotension and laryngeal or bronchial spasms and may be lethal if not managed properly. In addition, they result in the formation of localized edema and stimulation of sensory nerve endings leading to itching.[4]

D. Serotonin

Basophilic granules of mast cells, basophils, blood platelets, and enterochromaffin cells contain another biologically active mediator, serotonin or 5-hydroxytryptamine.[4] Upon activation or destruction, these cells release this hormone producing additional effects in anaphylactic reactions. The effects of serotonin include vasoconstriction at selected locations (particularly renal vessels), vasodilatation of muscular and cutaneous vessels, and stimulation of gastrointestinal and other smooth muscles. The role of this chemical mediator in anaphylaxis is overwhelmed by the effects of histamine and the exact implication of serotonin in this mechanism is not well understood.

E. Kinins

The relationship between kinin generation and allergic phenomena has been established.[5] When the polymorphonuclear cells phagocytize immune complexes, there is a release of a kinin-forming enzyme. The lesions produced in conditions like acute glomerulonephritis and rheumatoid arthritis may be a result of immune complex deposition where in turn the kinin liberation is possible. The kinins are very active biologically and produce vasodilatation, increased capillary permeability, edema, and stimulation of the sensory nerve endings. On a molar basis, the vasodilatation effect of kinins is nearly 10 times more potent than that of histamine. They also cause either a contraction or relaxation of a variety of smooth muscles in the body.

F. Prostaglandins

These chemicals are released in various tissues by the host cells by mechanical, chemical, or bacterial injuries. They are believed to be implicated in the inflammatory processes and are also found in arthritic joint fluids. Their presence during allergic reactions suggest that they may be involved in immunological injury.[6] Prostaglandins are also released by certain malignant growths. These chemicals have a number of diverse effects in different cells and tissues

III. ANAPHYLACTIC REACTIONS

The anaphylactic reactions are mediated through the release of biologically active substances from certain cells. In tissue, the mast cells, and in circulating blood, the basophils are involved. Eosinophils and blood platelets are also carriers of chemical mediators in anaphylaxis in some species. Nearly all chemicals described earlier may be involved in anaphylaxis, but histamine and another slow reacting substance are the most important ones.[7] The rate and amount of release of the chemical mediators determines the severity of symptoms and whether the reaction will be a generalized one or not. This release in turn depends on the amount of exposure and the degree of sensitization of the individual.[8] The last factor may be determined by history of prior exposure, genetic determinants, or by various environmental factors that are known to cause modification of immune responses.

The mechanism of anaphylactic reactions include the production of tissue-fixing antibodies called reagins. The reagin is a type of immunoglobulin, IgE, and binds to the cells or tissues through its Fc portion. There is some IgE present in circulating blood but it rarely indicates the amount of tissue-fixed antibody present in various cells. The release of biologically active mediators can be initiated by the reaction of specific antigens or anti-IgE antibodies reacting to cell-fixed reagin. The IgE can be skin-fixing, if it binds to the mast cells in skin and produces localized or generalized cutaneous anaphylaxis involving swelling or edema. Systemic anaphylaxis is produced by the reagin binding the circulatory cells and can be more serious since the effects of histamine resemble a parasympathetic stimulations. These involve smooth muscle contraction (including those in bronchi), increased vascular permeability, hypotension, slowing of heart, and increased pulmonary secretions. There is a decreased serum complement level associated with the systemic anaphylactic reaction.

Allergic reactions to natural antigens (e.g., food, pollen) are termed "atopic". The symptoms include asthma, hay fever, rhinitis, urticaria, conjunctivitis, eczema, or gastrointestinal reactions. The atopic allergic reactions are the same as the anaphylactic ones in their mechanisms.

IV. ARTHUS REACTION

This reaction, also known as *toxic-complex* reaction, can be caused either by the immunoglobulin directly reacting with the antigen in cells or by the formation of microprecipitates by soluble antigens and antibodies that are subsequently deposited on the walls of small blood vessels. The reaction leads to a local inflammation and requires complement fixation. The resultant accumulation of phagocytic cells and lysosome-releasing cells leads to the destruction of cells in the involved blood vessels. The reaction may occur in the lamina of arteries (serum sickness), renal glomerular basement vessels (glomerulonephritis), or in the cutaneous capillaries (typical arthus reaction). Certain other conditions like Goodpastures' syndrome, collagen disease, and amyloidosis are also caused by a similar mechanism.[9]

V. DELAYED HYPERSENSITIVITY REACTIONS

The delayed hypersensitivity reactions are the cell-mediated reactions and generally require no antibody. Specially sensitized lymphocytes are involved in this phenomenon. The reaction may involve either a direct destruction of target cells by the lymphocytes or the production of various lymphokines that may direct other cells for this function.[10] Examples of this reaction include cutaneous hypersensitivity as in tuberculin-type reactions, contact allergy, or graft-mediated responses. The antibody-dependent, cell-mediated cytolysis of target cells is carried on by IgG antibodies binding with these cells and the lymphocytes which have Fc receptors then attacking and causing the damage. The lymphocytes involved in this type of toxic reaction do not have membrane determinants for B or T cell markers and have been termed as K cells (killer lymphocytes).[11]

VI. ALLERGY TO CHEMICALS AND DRUGS

Any of the above pathologic mechanisms can be produced by hypersensitivity reactions involving small chemical molecules, which by themselves are not antigenic. These chemicals, or one of their transformation products within the body, may conjugate with serum or tissue proteins, and thus may become antigenic. Allergy to penicillin, for example is well known. Contact allergic mechanisms have been implicated in a substantial number of chemical or occupational dermatoses.

VII. AUTOIMMUNOLOGIC CONDITIONS

A number of autoallergic diseases have been described and their list is likely to grow as the causes of more diseases are discovered. Normally allergic reactions are not mounted against the normal tissue components. However, in certain conditions, either genetic or pathologic, the body can produce immune responses against its own tissues, particularly if the tissue proteins get access to the circulation or are altered as a result of injury or damage. It has been proposed that an inhibition of suppressor T cells may result in an unregulated clonal proliferation of B lymphocytes. For example, multiple thymus grafts have been able to protect the spontaneous autoallergic disease condition in genetically predisposed mice.[12]

In many cases autoimmunologic conditions are associated with the presence of autoantibodies specific against certain body tissues or their components. Detection of these autoantibodies has been a useful tool in the diagnosis of associated diseases. The antibodies present may be organ-specific or nonspecific in nature. In man, autoantibodies against a wide range of antigens such as nucleic acid, cell organelles, erythrocytes, platelets, and clotting factors have been described in systemic lupus erythematosus.[13] Some autoimmunologic conditions, however, may not show involvement of any of the autoantibodies, and sensitized T cells alone may be responsible for the production of tissue damage. There is increasing evidence that some autoallergic diseases are mediated via cellular mechanisms, e.g., autoallergic encephalomyelitis.

The autoallergic syndrome may be a possible explanation of the mechanisms involved in some immunotoxicological problems. Autoantibodies have been described in individuals exposed to a number of environmental chemicals (e.g., organophosphate insecticides). The tissue damage produced by such chemicals may be via initial modification of the normal tissue by chemicals resulting in the triggering of the autoimmune phenomenon against these tissues. If a number of immunocompetent cells are recruited for the production of autoantibodies or autoallergic cell-mediated mechanisms, there may be a significant alteration of the immune response of the individual against different invading antigens.

VIII. IMMUNODEFICIENCY AND IMMUNOTOXICOLOGICAL MECHANISMS

The description of various genetic disorders that lead to immunodeficiency is beyond the scope of this discussion. However, various immunodeficiency states are somewhat similar to those produced by exogenous chemicals. Table 2 summarizes selected possible sites where an alteration of the immune system is possible or has been observed. In many of the examples listed in Table 2, the exact location of action is still a matter of speculation and some of the mechanisms are hypothetical. These examples may only be used as illustrations of possible mechanisms or sites of immune action that have been investigated in previous studies.

Table 2
POSSIBLE IMMUNOTOXICOLOGICAL MECHANISMS AND IMMUNODEFICIENCY

Immunologic nature	Effect or mechanisms	Chemical agent or associated condition
General	Damage to primary lymphoid organs	Radiation, TCDD?
	Effect on stem cell producing site	Chloramphenicol, benzene, radiation
	Deficiency of polymorphonuclear leukocytes	Infections, chronic glomerulomatous disease, myeloperoxidase deficiency
	Inhibition of protein or nucleic acid synthesis	Antimetabolites, alkylating agents (cyclophosphamide)
	General stress mechanisms	Lack of nutrients, steroid hormones
Specific cellular	Interference with interactions between T cell and antigen	Cancer antigens, chronic infections
	Lack of specific lymphocytes (selective destruction)	Thymic aplastia, antilymphocytic serum
	Defective lymphocyte proliferation	Chronic infection
	Defective lymphokine production	Chronic mucocutaneous candidiasis
	Stimulation of T cells	Levamisole
Nonspecific Cellular	Maturation defect	(Hypothetical)
	Lack of lysozymes	Acute viral infection, steroids, phenothiazines
	Alteration of lymphocyte receptors	Alkylating agents (?)
Humoral	Absence of B lymphocytes	Specific antibodies to B cells; Bruton's sex-linked agammaglobulinemia
	Failure of differentiation to plasma cells	Defective antigen presentation, macrophage depression, lack of IgG and IgA with raised IgM.
Complement related	Deficiency or complement (notably C3)	Vinyl chloride, infections, tumors
	Complement activation	Transfusion reactions, erythroblastosis fetalis, hemolytic reactions to drugs or chemicals
Macrophage	Blockade of reticuloendothelial system	Saturating dose of carbon
	Macrophage stimulation	Adjuvant, endotoxin, *Listeria monocytogenes*
Enzyme inhibition	Inhibition of esterases	Organophosphates
	Stabilization of lysosomal membrane	(Hypothetical)
Immunotolerance or cellular anergy	Antigen-induced competition with recognition receptors	High dose of monomeric flagellin, tolerance to thyroglobulin
	Immune complex blocking factors	Certain tumor immunity
	Antibody induced immunosuppression	SRBC antibodies
Autoimmunologic	Production of antibodies or specific cells against normal tissues	Allergic encephalomyelitis, organ damage with specific antibodies

REFERENCES

1. **Gell, P. G. H., Coombs, R. R. A., and Lachmann, P. J.,** Classification of tissue-damaging allergic reactions, in *Clinical Aspects of Immunology,* 3rd ed., Blackwell Scientific, Oxford, 1975.
2. **Becker, E. L. and Henson, P. M.,** In vitro studies of immunologically induced secretions of mediators from cells and related phenomenon, *Adv. Immunol.,* 17, 94, 1973.
3. **Becker, E. L.,** Organophosphorus inhibitors and mechanisms of cell activation, in *Immunopharmacology,* Rosenthale, M. E. and Mansmann, H. C., Eds., Spectrum Publications, New York, 1975.
4. **Douglas, W. O.,** Autacoids, in *The Pharmacological Basis of Therapeutics,* Goodman, L. S. and Gilman, A., Eds., Macmillan, New York, 1975.
5. **Greenbaum, L. M.,** Kinins and immunity, in *Immunopharmacology* Rosenthale, M. E. and Mansmann, H. C., Eds., Spectrum Publications, New York, 1975.
6. **Tauber, A. I., Kaliner, M. A., Stechschulte, D. J., and Austen, K. F.,** Prostaglandins and the immunological release of chemical mediators from human lung, in *Prostaglandins and Cyclic AMP: Biological Actions and Clinical Applications,* Kahn, R. H. and Lands, W. E. M., Eds., Academic Press, New York, 1973.
7. **Block, K. S.,** The anaphylactic antibodies of mammals including man, *Prog. Allergy,* 10, 87, 1967.
8. **Sell, S.,** Atopic or anaphylactic reactions, in *Immunology, Immunopathology and Immunity,* 2nd ed., Harper and Row, Hagerstown, Md., 1975.
9. **Sell, S.,** Arthus (toxic complex) reactions, in *Immunology, Immunopathology and Immunity,* 2nd ed., Harper and Row, Hagerstown, Md., 1975.
10. **Cerottini, J. C. and Brunner, K. T.,** Cell mediated cytotoxicity, allograft rejection and tumor immunity, *Adv. Immunol.,* 18, 67, 1974.
11. **MacLennan, I. C. M. and Harding, B.,** Non-T cytotoxicity in vitro, in *Progress in Immunology II,* Brent, L. and Holbrough, J., Eds., North-Holland, Amsterdam, 1974.
12. **Kysela, S. and Steinberg, A. D.,** Increased survival of NZB/W mice given multiple syngeneic young thymus grafts, *Clin. Immunol. Immunopath.,* 2, 133, 1974.
13. **Spry, C. J. F.,** Autoallergic diseases, in *The Immune System,* Hobart, M, J. and McConnell, I., Eds., Blackwell Scientific, Oxford, 1975.

Chapter 6

PESTICIDES AND THE IMMUNE SYSTEM

Joseph C. Street

TABLE OF CONTENTS

I. INTRODUCTION

Pesticides constitute a unique group of biologically active chemicals in that they are produced for deliberate release into the environment, usually to produce some specific biocidal effect. Workers at all stages of pesticide formulation, manufacture, and application become exposed, at least on an occasional basis, while some experience routine exposure. Such exposures are chiefly by the dermal and respiratory routes. The general population is, in turn, exposed to the residues of pesticides, including their physical and biological degradation products, in air, water, and foods.

Man has acquired a little over three decades experience of exposure to the so-called "modern" organic pesticides since the introduction of DDT and DDT-related compounds in the 1940s. Epidemiologic review of that experience indicates that immune-system effects, including allergic dermatitis, are possibly the most frequent indications of toxic response to pesticides in their normal uses, while systemic poisoning or major chronic disease are noticably rare. The relative absence of the latter gives testimony to the general effectiveness of industrial and governmental regulatory controls upon pesticide manufacture and use, and to the associated public health surveillance based upon monitoring pesticide residues in agricultural products, foods, and drinking water. The toxicological testing of pesticides required in most countries to obtain permission for their marketing and use has not involved examination of possible effects upon the immune system beyond the evaluation of lymphoid tissues in the general pathology review. Recent strengthening of protocols in required premarketing toxicological assessments of pesticides will lessen risk of major disease, especially oncogenic disease, but will do little to identify the causes of immunotoxicity or to avert such effects.

This review is intended to survey the present knowledge of the immunotoxicity of pesticides, with commentary upon its public health significance and the continuing need for research. As will be readily seen, knowledge of pesticide immunotoxicology to date is largely descriptive with only modest beginnings toward understanding mechanisms underlying the effects. In most cases the effects have yet to be defined in immunological "state of the art" terms, and just as little is presently known about how these chemicals exert their effects. There is an equally great gap in perceiving any relationship between the structure of a chemical and its immunotoxic potential.

II. ALLERGIC RESPONSES TO PESTICIDES

Many pesticides have been associated with sensitizations producing allergic response. These cases are generally types of allergic dermatitis, often confirmed by the "patch test" technique. The citations in Table 1 indicate the wide spectrum of chemicals used as pesticides and associated with such sensitizations. The reports are primarily of the typical cell-mediated, inflammatory-response type involving mast cell depletion and characterized by erythema, edema and also eczema. They typically report cases of occupational exposure, frequently involving farmworkers. Apparently less frequent are specific IgE-dependent urticarial-type sensitivities, although these may be present upon repeated exposure with sensitive individuals. Many examples of pesticide-related photoallergy have been reported, but none has been thoroughly studied. A large proportion of these reports is from eastern Europe and Japan, a fact that probably attests more to the organization of public health surveillance and medical reporting in those countries than to unique sensitivity within their populations.

Several typical cases are summarized in the following paragraphs.

Nater et al.[20] described three cases of contact dermatitis caused by the fungicide, Maneb (manganese ethylenebisdithiocarbamate). Exposure related to its use in floriculture, with two of the subjects being affected in an office decorated with flowers and plants and the other in a flower shop. Patch tests not only confirmed Maneb as the allergen, but showed no cross-sensitivity to the zinc-containing analogue, zineb.

Contact with chrysanthemum plants that had been sprayed 2 hours previously with a mixture of the insecticide, Naled, the fungicide, Captan and the miticide, dicofol, caused several workers to experience burning and itching of the arms, face, neck, and abdomen.[13] The workers were cutting tops of unflowered plants, thus handling the plants with bare hands. Patch tests later established the sensitizing property of Naled (Dibrom, 1,2-dibromo-2,2-dichloroethyldimethyl phosphate). Sodium *N*-methyl dithiocarbamate (Nematin) used as a soil fumigant and seed potato treating agent has been associated with dermatitis.[21,32] This activity has been attributed to its hydrolytic product, methyl isothiocyanate. Circulating lymphocytes carrying Nematin recognition were demonstrated in sensitized individuals.[32]

Milby and Epstein reported finding six reactors from a group of 157 mosquito district workers plus 41 poultry ranchers accustomed to handling the insecticide malathion (*O*, *O*-dimethyl-*S*-diethylmercaptosuccinate-phosphorodithioate).[12] That frequency of sensitivity was low compared to their finding that nearly half of a group of male volunteers exhibited positive patch test responses to a dilute malathion solution 30 days following a skin application of 10% Malathion.

Nomura and his associates reported a frequency of 30 to 50% for dermatitis in men exposed to thiophanate-methyl [1,2-bis-(3-ethoxycarbonyl-2-thioureido) benzene] in citrus warehouse applications; rates in women were slightly greater.[16] These subjects suffered itching, redness, swellings, dry skin, and sometimes sensitized dermatitis as well as congestion of the ocular mucosa.

A number of clinical workers have observed photosensitization in pesticide-related dermatitis. Nomura[16] used a photo-patch test in assessing the role of pesticides in "lettuce dermatitis", Horiuchi and Ando similarly determined that paraquat, chlorothalomil, and trifluralin appear to produce a photoallergic dermatitis.[28] Peoples et al.[19] have reported that the clinical experience with captafol suggests that it is a primary irritant and probably a photosensitizing agent, responsible for several troublesome skin and eye injury cases in tomato-field workers.

The bulk of the reports listed in Table 1 are similar to these above. Clinically, pesticide effects do not appear to involve anaphylaxis. No evaluations of serum IgE in humans hypersensitive to pesticides have been reported, even though specific IgE levels have been shown to correlate with a number of other human allergies.

In laboratory animals, administration of certain pesticides has produced reactions characteristic of hypersensitivity. For example, the presence of IgE in serum of rats immunized intradermally with an albumin-conjugate of malathion has been demonstrated.[36]

Polychloropene, used as an insecticide in eastern Europe, has been shown to produce an immediate allergic reaction in sensitized guinea pigs.[37-39] It is a typical inflammatory-type reaction characterized by release of histamine, increased permeability and necrosis of vascular walls, and lymphoid infiltration. Subcutaneous, intravenous, and intratracheal sensitization of guinea pigs with thiram resulted in anaphylactic reactions when they were later challenged.[25] Thiram also produced contact dermatitis in rabbits upon intra- or epidermal administration.[40] Contact dermatitis was also observed in guinea pigs sensitized to thiram and several other dithiocarbamates, and to ethylene-bis-dithiocarbamates.[41] This is one of the few studies where chemical structure and toxicant activity were evaluated. The ethylene-bis-dithiocarbamates were found to be stronger sensitizers than the dimethyldithiocarbamates, and some cross-sensitivity was seen with the former

Table 1
REPORTS OF HUMAN DERMAL SENSITIVITY TO PESTICIDES

Insecticides	Ref.	Fungicides	Ref.
BHC	1	Benomyl	16, 1
Butyphos	2	Captan	8
Cartap	3	Difolatan	3, 4, 8, 17, 18, 19
Chlorfenvinphos	3		
Chlorobenzilate	4	Dinofen	9
Chlorophos	5	Mancozeb	8
Cyanox	3	Maneb	3, 16, 8, 20 21
Cyanphenphos	3		
DDT	6, 7	Nematin	21, 32
Diazinon	3, 4	PCNB	3
Dichlorvos	3, 8	Thiram	22, 23, 24, 25
Dicofol	8		
Dimite	8	Zineb	8, 3, 4, 26
Dinofen	9		
Fenitrothion	3, 4	**Herbicides**	**Ref.**
Formothion	3		
Karathane	10	CDAA	27
Leptophos	3	Chlorothalonil	8, 3, 4, 28, 16
Lindane	11		
Malathion	12	2, 4-D	29, 30, 31
Methomyl	3	Daconil	8
Methyl mercaptophos	2	Paraquat	8, 4, 28, 16
Naled	13	2, 4, 5-T	33, 34, 29, 31
Nicotine sulfate	8	Trifluralin	8, 3, 28, 16
Nitrofen	4, 14		
Omite	15	**Rodenticides**	**Ref.**
Ovex	8		
Phenthoate	3	Phosphine	35
Pirimiphos-methyl	9		
Salithion	8		
Schradan	2		
Thiometon	3		
Thiophanate	4, 16		

types.[41] Repeated intracutaneous injections or application to scarified skin were required to produce allergenic effects with paraquat in guinea pigs.[42]

With the wide scope of apparent allergic sensitization being produced by pesticides of many types, it is noteworthy that the lung seldom appears to be involved. Asthma-like morbidity is occasionally indicated in the epidemiologic surveys but seldom in case reports of pesticide sensitizations. This probably reflects nothing more than that under most instances of occupational exposure to pesticides,[44,45] the skin is far more heavily exposed than the airway, especially the deep lung.[44,45] In addition, the observed effects involve primarily local, nonsystemic effects, thus indicating weak IgE responses to these chemical sensitizers.

III. PESTICIDES AND AUTOIMMUNE DISEASE

Autoimmune responses, i.e., immune responses to body components, have been observed in exposed humans and animals dosed experimentally with some pesticides. Although autoimmune disease is rare, these experimental findings may indicate the need for more detailed appraisal of immune processes during premarket testing of new chemicals, including pesticides.

According to Katsenovich and Usmanova, liver autoantibodies were detected within a group of persons suffering with serious digestive or nervous disorders, and who had some history of contact with organochlorine and organophosphorus pesticides for periods of 2 to 20 years.[46] The appearance of autoantibodies was considered a significant, nonspecific indicator of early pathologic processes. That study, of course, provided only evidence of opportunity for pesticide association with the autoimmune process. A more temporal association with pesticides was reported by Kotlarek-Haus et al.,[47] involving a farmer requiring repeated hospitalization for hemolytic crises. His crises apparently coincided with the times of pesticide applications to his fields (DDT, lindane, fenthion, and 2,4-D) and were shown to involve anti-C gamma globulins in erythrocytes, a low complement titer, and positive direct Coombs test. Similarly, Brusilovskiy and coworkers[48] detected autoantibodies in patients exposed to caprolactam and methaphenilenediamine (*N,N*-dimethyl-N'-phenyl-N'-2-thenyl-ethylenediamine). These workers also found autoantibodies in guinea pigs sensitized with polychloropinene, thiram, and chlorophos (Trichlorophan, *O,O*-dimethyl-2,2,2-trichloro-1-hydroxy-ethylphosphonate).[48] The antibodies were tissue specific and correlated with the degree of tissue pathology observed. Antithyroid autoantibodies have been observed in rabbits with experimental bone fractures, but the titer of which was increased by butiphos treatment (*S,S,S,*-tributyl-phosphorotrithioate),[49] and antihepatic, -kidney, -stomach, and -intestine reacting antibodies were detected in goats dosed with the pesticides Anthio® and Milbex[50] (dicofol with 4-chlorophenyl-2,4,5-trichlorophenyl azosulfide). Hexachlorocyclohexane (BHC) and methyl–mercaptophos, when administered repeatedly to rabbits resulted in autoantibodies against both liver and kidney tissue.[51]

Similar findings were reported from mice and rats dosed repeatedly with methyl–mercaptophos, phosphamide, aldrin, or monuron.[52] Antihepatic autoantibodies were first detected on the 7th day of dosing and reached a maximum by the 30th day.

The development of liver autoimmunity has been studied in experimental carbon tetrachloride poisoning (itself a fumigant pesticide).[53] Antihepatic antibodies occurred in relation to the degree of dose-dependent interlobular necrosis.

These reports, most of which could not be reviewed in the original, complete form, indicate a considerable potential for autoimmune reactions associated with pesticide exposure. Most, however, imply that effects accompany the development of substantial tissue pathology, either as cause or effect. Regardless, it serves to indicate that autoimmune reactions are probably quite dose-dependent and, therefore, unlikely to become manifest as low dosage phenomena. Nevertheless, this appears to be an important, but seriously neglected, topic for research.

IV. PESTICIDE EFFECTS ON HOST DEFENSES

A fully responsive immunologic system is essential for protection against encounters with toxins and infectious agents and organisms. The response of the host to a pathogenic microorganism, for example, is a complex process involving phagocytosis, antigen processing, expression of immune resistance via phagocytic components, participation of the reticuloendothelial system, and the utilization of complement, antibody, and cell-mediated factors. The response may be altered by many different mechanisms resulting in varied resistance of the host to the pathogen. That chemical toxicants may contribute to altered host defenses is not unappreciated, yet this has not been a topic of much active interest within the field of toxicology. Nevertheless, recent investigations have shown that many pesticides produce altered host defense following suitable dosing. Again, the present understanding of these effects is largely at the descriptive level and very little of the research has been directed to mechanisms, or to development of unifying concepts.

Much of the available literature has been summarized in Table 2, which lists the pesticides by the usual classes, the species observed, dosing rate and schedule, and the general effects observed. Both stimulation and suppression of the immune response are observed, often with the same agent during a single experiment. In fact, such a biphasic effect, seems fairly general during short term experiments.

V. EFFECTS ON HUMORAL RESPONSES

Early work by Wassermann and his associates with DDT, dieldrin, and lindane helped to establish the fact of the effects of these pesticides upon body defenses.[59-61] Rats ingesting p,p′-DDT showed increased liver weight, depressed antiovalbumin titers, and lowered gamma globulin serum concentrations. Wassermann's group also showed a decreased antisalmonella titer in rabbits dosed with DDT. Similarly, rats treated with lindane or dieldrin showed a reduced response of the 7s fraction of serum gamma globulin after *Salmonella typhii* administration.[59] Others obtained somewhat similar results in chickens administered DDT or Mirex®, which produced reduced activity of bursal, splenic, and thymic lymphocytes from chickens.[65] IgG levels were simultaneously reduced but IgM levels were elevated.

Carbamates and organophosphates were also found to cause similar altered humoral response. For example, Street and Sharma[88] reported dose-related alteration of the immune response in rabbits treated with DDT, a PCB (Aroclor 1254®), carbaryl, carbofuran, or methyl parathion. These treatments resulted in decreased counts of activated lymphocytes in lymph nodes, in reduction of germinal centers in the spleen, in increased atrophy of the thymus cortex, and decreased antigen-induced gamma globulin; some variations in these effects were seen among the chemicals. Follow up study in mice dosed with carbofuran established that IgG, IgG_{2A}, and IgG_{2B} levels were markedly depressed; IgA and IgM levels were not greatly affected.[77] Only IgG_{2B} was appreciably reduced by methyl parathion. The dosed mice were also deficient in gamma globulin compared to controls.[77]

The immunobiological indicators were found to be considerably more sensitive than the biochemical indexes of toxicity when these were compared in rats and rabbits given trichlorfon, carbetox, or BHC.[89] Treatments with malathion, DDVP, and lindane were shown to suppress agglutination in rabbits given *S. typhii* vaccine.[75] When the effects of several widely used pesticides of different types on the primary immune response were studied, Wiltrout et al.[90] noted that each had the potential to suppress an ongoing primary humoral response when administered at a single high dose, as measured by the number of antibody plaque-forming cells in spleen. However, repeated dosing with these chemicals for 8 or 28 days, respectively, prior to immunization had no significant effect upon the plaque-forming cell response, except for the case of parathion. This illustrates the importance of the temporal factors in exposure to both chemical and antigen in such experimentation.

Failure to understand and appreciate the importance of dosage schedules as well as the timing of immune sensitization and challenge probably accounts for much of the variability found in this literature. The data in Table 3 and Figure 1 illustrate two aspects of time-related variability in response. The humoral response to bacteriophage in DDT-pretreated rabbits (Table 3) was seen to lag that of controls; however, by the third and fourth week the antibody titers were similar.[91] Thus, observing the "effect" depended upon the time of observation. In contrast, the host defense by mice treated with carbofuran in the diet for varying times was seen to diminish with increasing

Table 2
EFFECTS OF PESTICIDES UPON HOST DEFENSE MECHANISMS

Pesticide	Species	Treatment or exposure	Effects	Ref.
		Chlorinated insecticides		
Dieldrin	Rabbits	Drinking water, 50 ppm	Reduced response of the 7s fraction serum gamma globulin (with *Salmonella typhi*)	54
		3 months	Slight reduction in IgG fraction of gamma globulins after 1 and 2 months; rise in albumin in first month	55
	Mallard duck	Dietary, 20, 40 ppm	Treated ducks challenged with duck hepatitis virus died over a longer period of time than untreated ducks; mortality of treated ducks was higher	56
	L-Moore cells of human lymphocytoid origin	12.5 mg/mℓ of log phase culture (LD_{50})	High frequencies of chromosomal breaks and exchanges	57
Lindane	Mouse	Dietary, 167 ppm 6 weeks	Enhanced sensitivity to the lethal effects of endotoxin and malarial parasite suggest a significantly impaired host-defense	58
p, p′ DDT	Rat	Drinking water 200 ppm 35 days	30% decrease in an antiovalbumin antibodies rise in serum albumin and decrease in serum globulin fractions	59
	Rabbit	Drinking water 200 ppm 38 days	Decrease in antibody titer, total, and 7s 8 globulins (with *Salmonella*)	60
	Rat and rabbit	0.5 mg/kg 1.0 mg/kg chronic	Decrease in phagocytic activity of leukocytes, antibodies formation, protective properties of the serum	64

Table 2 (continued)
EFFECTS OF PESTICIDES UPON HOST DEFENSE MECHANISMS

Pesticide	Species	Treatment or exposure	Effects	Ref.
		Chlorinated insecticides		
p, p′ DDT	Rat	4 months	Inhibition of *Typhus abdominalis* antibody formation most pronounced during initial phase of immunization; effect of chlorophos and DDT carbamates; possible stimulation of antibody formation during final stage of immunogenesis	62
	Chicken	Oral, alternate days 10, 30, 50 mg/kg 8—38 days of age	DDT may have affected the development of immunity to histomoniasis — pathologic lesions observed at all levels	63
DDT	Rabbit	Drinking water 200 ppm 35 days	Impaired immunological responses in *Salmonella* treated rabbits but not with sheep red blood cell antigens; suggests that immunological response is inversely proportional to amount of total DDT in plasma	61
	Chicken	Dietary 100—400 ppm	At 400 ppm, withdrawal of feed for 3—4 days before BSA injection significantly reduced precipitan production and IgG levels; withdrawal of feed for seven days after BSA injection significantly reduced titers	65
Mirex	Chicken	Dietary, 200—800 ppm up to 5 weeks of age	Significant depression in levels of IgG and IgM; 500 ppm	65
	Chicken lymphocytes		IgG levels significantly reduced, IgM levels markedly elevated; no significant difference in total antibody production	66
Hexachloro-benzene	Male rat	Dietary, 250 ppm 8—10 weeks	Decreased rosette formation of alveolar macrophages at fixed antibody conc	67

	Mouse	Dietary, 167 ppm 6 weeks	Impared immunological responsiveness — lower primary serum IgA, decreased primary and secondary splenic antibody plaque-forming cell; no change in size, number, or cellular populations of spleen germinal follicles	68
	Mouse	Dietary	Enhanced sensitivity to the lethal effects of endotoxin and malarial parasite	58
Heptachlor	Chicken	Dietary 1 ppm 3—8 weeks of life	Increased by (28%) weight of the bursa of Fabricius	69
Endrin	Human lymphocytes	10μM	Inhibition of stimulation by phytohemagglutinin	70
DDT	Mice	Painted on the abdomen of young mice 11 days	Highest mortality due to EMC virus in group exposed to solvent + emulsifier; Fenitrothion appeared to protect mice but DDT may partially counteract protective effect	71
		Organophosphorus insecticides		
Leptophos	Mouse	Dietary 10, 100, 500 ppm 12 weeks	No significant alteration in primary and secondary immune responses as measured by hemolytic plaque assay of antibody forming cells	72
Ronnel	Chicken	Dietary 0.5, 1.0 ppm 3—8 weeks of life	Weight of the Bursa of Fabricius increased 39% (l ppm) and 49% (0.5 ppm)	69
Triisopropyl-phosphate	Rabbit	0.5 to 8 m*M*, in vitro	Inhibition of locomotion of polymorphonuclear leukocytes	73
Dimethoate	Rat Mouse	Single dose LD_{50} Chronic admin.	Decreased no. of immunocomplementary cells of the spleen and the hemagglutinin titer in the serum; stimulation of antibody production followed by depression.	74
DEP	Rabbit	0.5 to 8 m*M*, in vitro	Inhibition of locomotion of polymorphonuclear leukocytes	73
Dichlorvos	Rabbit		Suppressed agglutination (rabbits exposed to *S. typhi* vaccine)	75

Table 2 (continued)
EFFECTS OF PESTICIDES UPON HOST DEFENSE MECHANISMS

Pesticide	Species	Treatment or exposure	Effects	Ref.
		Organophosphorus insecticides		
Carbophenothion	Human lymphocytes	10 μM	Inhibition of stimulation by phytohemagglutinin	70
Crufomate	Human lymphocytes	10 μM	Inhibition of stimulation by phytohemagglutinin	70
Trichlorofon	Guinea Pig	In vivo and in vitro	Significant decreases in activity of guinea pig complement	76
		Intramuscular	Inhibition preceded by increased complement activity	
Methyl-parathion	Human lymphocytes	10 μM	Inhibition of stimulation by phytohemagglutinin	70
	Mouse	Dietary, 0.08, 3.0 mg/kg/day; 4 weeks	Upon challenge dose of *S. typhimurium* C_5' cells, dose-related increase in mortality in unvaccinated mice and protection by immunization was decreased; increased mortality was associated with increased numbers of viable bacteria in blood, decreased total gamma globulins and specific immunoglobins in serum, and reduced splenic blast transformation in response to mitogens	77
	Rat		Marked reaction of typhoid group of agglutinins, animals immunized by polyvaccines	78
Methyl-mercaptophos	Rat	Single dose, LD_{50}	Decreased number of immunocomplementary cells of spleen and the hemagglutinin titer in the serum	74
	Mouse	Chronic admin.	Stimulation of antibody production followed by depression	
Malathion	Rabbit		Suppressed agglutination (rabbits exposed to *S. typhi* vaccine)	75

		Carbamate insecticides		
Carbofuran	Mouse	Dietary, 0.1, 0.6, 1.0 mk/kg/day, 4 weeks	Upon challenge dose of *S. typhimurium* C_5' cells dose-related increase in mortality in unvaccinated mice and protection by immunization was decreased; increased mortality was associated with increased numbers of viable bacteria in blood, decreased total gamma globulins and specific immunoglobins in serum, and reduced splenic blast transformation in response to mitogens; serum opsonin activity was slightly reduced	77
Carbamates	Rat	4 months	Inhibition of *Typhus abdominalis* antibody formation most pronounced during initial phase of immunization; effect of chlorophos and DDT is greater than carbamates; possible stimulation of antibody formation during final stage of immunogenesis	62
Dicresyl	Rat	Dietary, 20 mg/kg 5 times per week, 4, 5 months	Reduction in nonspecific immunity; reduction in infection resistance against *E. Coli* and *Staphylococcus;* impairment in cellular and humoral immunity	79
Carbaryl	Rat	Oral, 400 mg/kg single dose	Reduction in immunological reactivity for more than 2 weeks; disturbances in the humoral, cellular, and barrier indices regarding the beta-lysin and lysoyzme levels, serum complement activity, percentages of active neutrophils, phagocytosis and digestion indices	80
	Rat	Dietary, 36 mg/kg 5 times per week, 4, 5 months	Reduction in nonspecific immunity; reduction in infection resistance against *E. coli* and *Staphylococcus.* Impairment in cellular and humoral immunity	79
	Rat	Oral in vegetable oil 1/20 to 1/5 LD_{50}; 70 or 120 days	Antibody development (vs. typhoid) decreased as dose increased	81

Table 2 (continued)
EFFECTS OF PESTICIDES UPON HOST DEFENSE MECHANISMS

Pesticide	Species	Treatment or Exposure	Effects	Ref.
		Carbamate insecticides		
Carbaryl	Rats	Oral 1/20—1/5 LD_{50}	Inhibition of immunity to tetanus toxoid, 1/5 and 1/10 LD_{50}	82
	Rat Rabbit	20 mg/kg	Decrease in phagocytic activity of leukocytes and antibody formation	64
	Female rat	Oral, daily 2 mg/kg 9 months	Significant decrease in agglutinin titers during early stages. Inhibition of phagocytic activity of neutrophils; reduced complement activity of blood serum; slight decrease in spleen immunoblast level, dystrophic changes in spleen-sinusal endothelium and decreased neutrophilic and eosinophilic leukocytes	83
	Rat	Oral 1.5 mg/kg/day 6 months	Significant decrease in the size of the lymphatic follicles in the spleen	84
		Miticides		
Milbex	Goat	Gastric tube 320, 620, 940, 1,400, 1,750 mg/kg single dose	Inhibited antibody formation and phagocytic activity of the neutrophilic leukocytes; circulating liver, kidney, stomach, and intestine autoantibodies detected in serum during first 2 months after poisoning	85
	Goat	Dietary 2.1, 4.2, and 21.0 mg/kg 90 days	Increased immunogenesis during the first 30 to 45 days; subsequent inhibition and lowered agglutinin titers; steady inhibition of phagocytic activity of neutrophils, autoimmune processes indicated by the presence of autoantibodies in the blood	50

Chloro- benzilate	Rat	Single dose, LD_{50}	Decreased number of immunocomplementary cells of the spleen, lowered hemagglutinin titer	74
		Chronic admin.	Stimulation of antibody production followed by depression	74
		Herbicides		
Fluometuron	Rat	Single dose, LD_{50}	Decreased number of immunocomplementary cells of the spleen and the hemagglutinin titer in the serum	74
	Mouse	Chronic admin.	Stimulation of antibody production followed by depression	
Diquat	Rat	10^{-6} mol/ℓ and higher conc.	Irreversible damage at in vitro conc. as low as 10^{-6} mol/ℓ; peritoneal and alveolar macrophages	86
	Mouse	10^{-5} mol/ℓ and higher conc.	Reduction in cloning efficiency at 10^{-5} mol/ℓ; irreversible damage at higher conc., in vitro	
Paraquat	Rat	10^{-6} mol/ℓ and higher conc.	Irreversible damage at in vitro conc. as low as 10^{-6} mol/ℓ; peritoneal and alveolar macrophages	86
Linuron	Rat	Oral 8 mg/kg/day 6 months	Significant decrease in the size of the lymphatic follicles in the spleen	84
Monum	Rat	Single dose, LD_{50}	Decreased no. of immunocomplementary cells of the spleen and the hemagglutinin titer in the serum	74
	Mouse	Chronic admin.	Stimulation of antibody production followed by depression	

Table 2 (continued)
EFFECTS OF PESTICIDES UPON HOST DEFENSE MECHANISMS

Pesticide	Species	Treatment or exposure	Effects	Ref.
		Carbamate Herbicides		
Tillam	Rat	Oral, 750 mg/kg, single dose	Reduction in immunological reactivity for more than two months; disturbances in the humoral, cellular, and barrier indices regarding the beta-lysin and lysozyme levels, serum complement activity, percentages of active neutrophils, phagocytosis, and digestion indices	80
		Dietary 56 mg/kg 5 times per week, 4.5 months	Reduction in nonspecific immunity; reduction in resistance against *E. coli* and *Staphylococcus* infection; impairment in cellular and humoral immunity	79
Molinate	Rat	Dietary, 33 mg/kg 5 times per week, 4.5 months	Reduction in nonspecific immunity; reduction in resistance against *E. coli* and *Staphylococcus* infection; impairment in cellular and humoral immunity	79
Propham	Human lymphocytes	10 μM	Slight inhibition of lymphocyte stimulation in vitro by phytohemagglutinin	70
Barban	Rat	Dietary, 200 mg/kg, single dose	Disturbances in the humoral, cellular, and barrier indices regarding the beta-lysin and lysozyme levels, serum complement activity, percentages of active neutrophils, phagocytosis, and digestion indexes	80
	Rat	Dietary, 26 mg/kg 5 times per week, 4.5 months	Reduction in nonspecific immunity; reduction in resistance against *E. coli* and *Staphylococcus* infection; impairment in cellular and humoral immunity	79

		Fungicides		
Triphenyltin Acetate	Guinea pig	Dietary, 15 ppm 49, 77, 104 days	Decreased immunologic response (tetanus toxoid), decrease in immunologically active cells in popliteal lymph nodes after 104 days	87
Zineb	Rat Rabbit	Oral, 100 mg/kg—500 mg/kg, chronic	Decrease in phagocytic activity of leukocytes, antibody formation	64
	Rat	Oral, daily 10 mg/kg 9 months	Significant decrease in agglutinin titers during early stages; reduced complement activity of blood serum; slight decrease in spleen immunoblast level; dystrophic changes in spleen-sinusal endothelium and decreased neutrophilic and eosinophilic leukocytes	83
	Rat	Oral, 12.5, 125 mg/kg/day 6 months	Significant decrease in the size of the lymphatic follicles in the spleen	84
Ziram	Rat	Oral, daily 2.5 mg/kg 9 months	Significant decrease in agglutinin titers during early stages. Inhibition of phagocytic activity of neutrophils; reduced complement activity of blood serum; slight decrease in spleen-sinusal endothelium and neutrophilic and eosinophilic leukocytes	83
Eptam	Rat	Oral, 1,000 mg/kg; single dose	Disturbances in the humoral, cellular, and barrier indices regarding the beta-lysin and lysozyme levels, serum complement activity, percentages of active neutrophils, phagocytosis and digestion indices; reduction in immunological reactivity for one week	80
	Rat	Dietary, 84 mg/kg 5 times per week 4, 5 months	Reduction in nonspecific immunity; reduction in infection resistance against *E. coli* and *Staphylococcus;* impairment in cellular and humoral immunity	79

Table 2 (continued)
EFFECTS OF PESTICIDES UPON HOST DEFENSE MECHANISMS

Pesticide	Species	Treatment or exposure	Effects	Ref.
		Fungicides		
Maneb	Rat	Oral, daily 0.75 mg/kg 9 months	Significant decrease in agglutinin titers during early stages; slight decrease in spleen immunoblast level; dystrophic changes in spleen-sinusal endothelium and reduced neutrophilic and eosinophilic leukocytes	83
	Rat	Oral, 1,000 mg/kg single dose	Disturbances in the humoral cellular and barrier indices regarding the beta-lysin and lysozyme levels, serum complement activity, percentages of active neutrophils, phagocytosis, and digestion indices; reduction in immunological reactivity for one week	80
	Rat	Dietary 150 mg/kg 5 times per week 4, 5 months	Reduction in nonspecific immunity; reduction in infection resistance against *E. coli* and *Staphylococcus;* impairment in cellular and humoral immunity	79
Thiram	Rat Rabbit	0.5 mg/kg 1.0 mg/kg chronic	Decrease in phagocytic activity of leukocytes, antibody formation, and protective properties of the serum	64
	Rat	Oral 400 mg/kg single dose	Disturbances in the humoral, cellular and barrier indices regarding the beta-lysin and lysozyme levels, serum complement activity, percentages of active neutrophils, phagocytosis, and digestion indices; reduction in immunological reactivity for more than 2 months	80
	Rat	Dietary 37 mg/kg 5 times per week 4, 5 months	Reduction in nonspecific immunity; reduction in infection resistance against *E. coli* and *Staphylococcus;* impairment in cellular and humoral immunity	79

Table 3
ANTIBODY TITERS TOWARD BACTERIOPHAGE T_4 DEVELOPED IN CONTROL AND DDT-TREATED RABBITS

		Bleeding period		
Treatment	Preantigen	Antigen + 14 days	Antigen + 21 days	Antigen + 28 days
Control	0	3.8 ± 1.3	4.5 ± 1.2	5.3 ± 1.1
DDT, 100 ppm in feed	0	2.0 ± 0.4	4.3 ± 0.5	4.5 ± 0.6

Note: Immunization by bacteriophage injection i.m. after rabbits had been consuming DDT-treated feed for 8 weeks; DDT feeding continued throughout the remaining 4 week experimental period. The values represent titer values expressed as the exponent in the series of serial dilutions of serum designated as 1/2n (mean ± S.E.); thus a value of 5 indicates a titer of $1/2^5$ or 1/32.

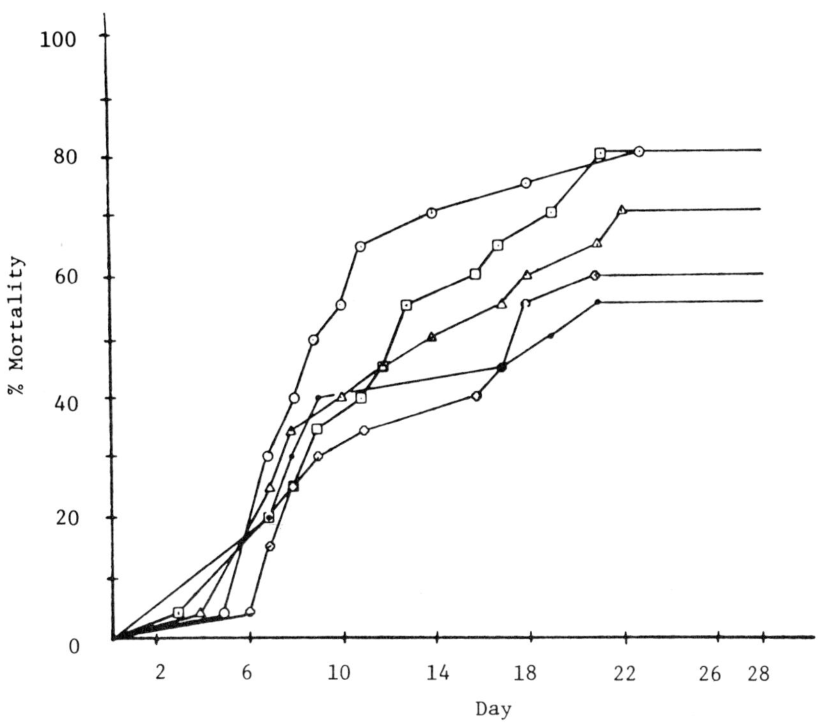

FIGURE 1. Cumulative mortality in mice treated with carbofuran for different time lengths and challenged with 1 × 10 *S. typhimurium* C'_5 Data from Fan.[92] Key: • Control; ◇ 1 week; △ 2 weeks; □ 3 weeks; ○ 4 weeks; all data given in 1 mg C∓/kg/day (From Fan, A., Ph.D. dissertation, Utah State University, Logan, 1980.)

duration of the pesticide treatment (Figure 1).[77] Again, the time of observation was a determinant of the effect.

These observations direct attention to the probabliity of toxicant effects being produced at the level of those lymphoid cells involved in antigen processing and antibody formation.

Limited observations, some made with pesticides and some with related chemicals such as TCDD, PCB, and vinyl chloride, support the premise that these chemicals act, at least in part, to inhibit the development and function of immunogenic lymphocytes.

VI. EFFECTS ON PHAGOCYTIC CELLS

A number of the studies listed in Table 2 were conducted with a challenge injection of a pathogen; the ensuing infection was then evaluated in various ways including the mortality rates. Such tests obviously involve several aspects of host defense, yet phagocytic activity is a key function in the process. The work of Olefir[79,80] showed increased infectivity of *Escherichia coli* and *Staphlococcus* in rats fed certain carbamate insecticides (e.g., carbaryl) and thiocarbamate fungicides (e.g., eptam and maneb). This was accompanied by altered nonspecific immunity seen as decreases in serum complement level, phagocytic index, percentage of active neutrophils, and as the bactericidal activity of serum and skin, and also as increased bacterial counts in tissues. Similar experiments demonstrating enhanced susceptibility to infection have been reported for a wide variety of pesticides and related substances.[56,68,64,77,81] Fan[78] obtained evidence from mice under dietary treatment with carbofuran and methyl parathion that these pesticides enhanced sensitivity to *Salmonella typhimurium* infection in both naive and immunized animals. Bacterial clearance rates from the circulation were retarded, and evidence was obtained that phagocytic activities were altered as well as bacteriocidal properties. There was also indication of reduced opsonin levels. These findings were complemented by the observed decrease in IgG_2 that is likely involved in opsonization and phagocyte activation processes.

VII. PESTICIDE EFFECTS ON CELL-MEDIATED IMMUNITY

Pesticide interactions with cell-mediated immune processes have received relatively little direct attention. However, several studies give evidence that T cell-dependent processes are subject to alteration under appropriate conditions of pesticide exposure. Olefir,[79,80] for example, demonstrated impairment in rats receiving single or long-term dosing with carbamate insecticides. Similarly, Street and Sharma[88] reported effects upon the thymus, reduced tuberculin sensitivity, and other indicators of cellular immune reactivity in pesticide-treated rabbits.

Tissue graft experiments in animals under pesticide treatment have not appeared. However, experimentation with tumor cell transplants involving other chemical stressors suggest that cell-mediated immune processes are quite responsive.

VIII. SUMMARY

Interactions of environmental chemicals (such as pesticides with the immune system and host defenses) appear common enough to have potential impact on public health. This is recognized in some countries, but generally the public health authorities are not alerted to these possibilities, except when patients present hypersensitivity-related complaints. As pointed out by Adkinson[93], the resiliency of the immune system is great, and undoubtedly this applies to stress by environmental chemicals. Nevertheless, study of the effect of chronic exposure to low levels of pesticides and other environmental chemicals on immune responses should be pursued. Agents showing indications of selective toxicity for the immune system and evaluation of the clinical consequences of increased susceptibility to infection should receive particular attention, as should consideration of the status of immune surveillance with respect to the incidence of cancers.

REFERENCES

1. **Yamamoto, K., Kinoshita, K., and Uchihira, T.,** A case of secondary erythroderma possibly due to BHC, *Karute,* 6, 61, 1973.
2. **Mirakhmedov, U. M. and Yusupov, B. Y.,** Clinical aspects of dermatoses caused by poisonous chemicals in agricultural workers, *Gig. Tr. Prof. Zabol.,* 17, 48, 1973.
3. **Kambe, Y., Ide, T., and Takeshige, M.,** Investigation on allergy due to pesticides by patch test II, *Nippon Noson Igakkai Zasshi,* 25, 628, 1976.
4. **Hanada, K., Kameda, T., Suzuki, Y., Kayashi, S., Ohagi, A., and Sugaya, H.,** An investigation of patch test dermatitis. IV. A comparison between farmers and non-farmers, *Akita-Ken Noson Igakkai Zasshi,* 23, 6, 1977.
5. **Polyak, N. R.,** Immunoserological and immunocytological reactions in response to sensitization with some pesticides, *Gig. Tr. Prof. Zabol.,* 5, 14, 1974.
6. **Vanat, S. V. and Vanat, I. M.,** Contributions to the toxic-allergic reaction induced by DDT, *Klin. Med.,* 49, 126, 1971.
7. **Mirakhmedov, U. M. and Karimov, A. M.,** The effect of pesticides on the skin of agricultural workers, *Vestn, Dermatol. Venerol.,* 16, 50, 1972.
8. **Horiuchi, N., Kambe, Y., Kato, E., Ando, S., and Yanagisawa, T.,** Studies on diagnostic standards on dermatitis due to pesticides. IV. Investigation on lettuce growing farmers, *Nippon Noson Igakki Zasshi,* 26, 566, 1977.
9. **Bainova, A., Nesheva, S., and Tsonevski, D.,** Contact dermatitis in vegetable hot-house workers, *Dermatol. Venerol. (Sofia),* 17, 85, 1978.
10. **Mazzella di Bosco, M.,** Some cases of occupational poisoning with dinitrophenols (binapacryl, DNOC, Karathane) in agricultural workers, *Eur. J. Toxicol.,* 3, 325, 1970.
11. **Schmid, R.,** Cutaneous porphyria in Turkey, *N. Engl. J. Med.,* 263, 397, 1960.
12. **Milby, T. H. and Epstein, W. L.,** Allergic contact sensitivity to malathion, *Arch. Environ. Health,* 9, 434, 1964.
13. **Edmundson, W. F. and Davies, J. E.,** Occupational dermatitis from naled, *Arch. Environ. Health,* 15, 89, 1967.
14. **Nomura, S.,** Studies on the diagnostic standards of dermatitis due to pesticides for agricultural uses, *Nippon Noson Igakkai Zasshi,* 26, 49, 1977.
15. **Nishioki, K., Kozuka, T., and Tashiro, M.,** Dermatitis by agricultural miticide, *Skin Res.,* 12, 15, 1970.
16. **Nomura, S., Matsushita, T., Arimatsu, T., and Tomio, T.,** Results of health examination on persons applying organosulfur fungicides, Report of studies commissioned by the Ministry of Health and Welfare, *Jpn. Soc. Rural Med.,* 25, 36, 1976.
17. **Groundwater, J. R.,** Difolatan dermatitis in a welder; non-agricultural exposure, *Contact Derm.,* 3, 104, 1977.
18. **Takamatsu, M., Futatsuka, M., Arimatsu, Y., Maeda, H., Inuzuka, T., and Takamatsu, S.,** Epidemiologic survey on dermatitis from a new fungicide used in tangerine orchards in Kumamoto prefecture, *J. Kumamoto Med. Sci.,* 42, 854, 1968.
19. **Peoples, S. A., Maddy, K. T., Tochilin, S., and Edmiston, S.,** Human health problems associated with exposure to the fungicide Captafol (difolatan) in California, *Vet. Human Toxicol.,* 20, 184, 1978.
20. **Nater, J. P., Terpstra, H., and Bleumink, E.,** Allergic contact sensitization to the fungicide Maneb, *Contact Derm.,* 5, 24, 1976.
21. **Matsushita, T., Arimatsu, N., and Tomio, T.,** Experimental studies on the onset of allergic dermatitis due to dithiocarbamate pesticides, *Nippon Kogyo Eisei Gakkai Nenkai Hokoku,* 49, 40, 1976.
22. **Baer, R. L. and Rosenthal, S. A.,** The germicidal action on human skin of soap containing tetramethylthiuram disulfide, *J. Invest. Dermatol.,* 23, 193, 1954.
23. **Blank, I. H.,** Allergic hypersensitivity to an antiseptic soap, *JAMA,* 160, 1225, 1956.
24. **Kligman, A. M.,** The identification of cantact allergens by human assay, *J. Invest. Dermatol.,* 47, 393, 1966.
25. **Brusilovskiy, Y. S. and Fialkovskiy, A. M.,** Experimental study of the effect of thiram administration on various allergic reactions, *Gig. Tr. Prof. Zabol.,* 17, 52, 1973.
26. **Zorin, P. M.,** Allergic dermatitis from zineb, *Vestn. Dermatol. Venerol.,* 44, 65, 1970.
27. **Spencer, M.,** Herbicide dermatitis, *JAMA,* 198, 1307, 1966.
28. **Horiuchi, N. and Ando, S.,** Clinical symptoms of dermatitis due to pesticides, especially its relationship with sunlight dermatitis, *Nippon Noson Igakkai Zasshi,* 26, 87, 1977.
29. **Poland, A. P., Smith, D., Metter, G., and Possick, P.,** A health survey of workers in a 2,4-D and 2,4,5-T plant, *Arch. Environ. Health,* 22, 316, 1971.
30. **Balo-Banga, M. J., Antoni, F., Altmann, H., Vinecze, I., and Kocsis, F.,** Case report: Bullous dermatitis after exposure to 2,4-D, *Ber. Oesterr. Studienges. Atomenerge,* 2218, 1, 1973.

31. **Jung, H. D. and Wolfe, F.,** Contact eczema due to Selest 100 herbicides in forestry, *Dtsch. Gesundheitswes.*, 32, 1464, 1977.
32. **Schubert, H.,** Contact dermatitis to sodium N-methyldithiocarbamate, *Contact Derm.*, 4, 380, 1978.
33. **Fetisov, M. I.,** Occupational hygiene in work with herbicides in the 2,4-D group, *Gig. Sanit.*, 31, 28, 1966.
34. **Bikbulatova, L. I. and Telegrina, K. A.,** Clinical aspects of skin lesions occurring with the production of the butyl ester of 2,4,5-trichlorophenoxy-acetic acid, *Tr. Ufim. Nauchno-Issled. Inst. Gig. Profzabol.*, 4, 215, 1968.
35. **Akoboshi, S., Takahashi, M., Seki, K., Kameda, S., Tashiro, M., and Harada, A.,** A case of acute phosphine toxicosis with chronic course, *Jpn. Assoc. Ind. Health*, 50, 285, 1977.
36. **Vijay, H. M., Mendoza, C. E., and Lavergne, G.,** Production of homocytotropic antibodies (IgE) to malathion in the rat, *Toxicol. Appl. Pharmacol.*, 44, 137, 1978.
37. **Viyevskaya, N. A. and Makovskaya, E. I.,** Study of the allergenic properties of polychloropinene, *Vrach. Delo*, 4, 132, 1973
38. **Viyevasky, N. A. and Baida, N. A.,** Study of pathochemical stages of allergic reaction to polychloropinene, *Vrach. Delo*, 4, 121, 1974.
39. **Viyevskaya, N. A.,** Histological examination of organs after combined exposure to polychloropinene and alcohol, *Vrach. Delo*, 8, 119, 1973.
40. **Brusilovsky, E. S. and Fialkovsky, A. M.,** Experimental study of the dermato-allergic effect of thiram, *Vestn. Dermatol. Venerol.*, 47, 28, 1973.
41. **Matsushita, T., Yoshioka, M., Nomura, S., and Arimatsu, T.,** Relation between the chemical structure of dithiocarbamate fungicides and the appearance of contact allergy, *Nippon Eiseigaku Zasshi*, 32, 201, 1977.
42. **Fodre, Z., Sipos, K., and Berencsi, G.,** Study of the irritating and allergenic effects of Gramoxone in guinea pigs, *Egeszsegtudomany*, 21, 244, 1978.
43. **Hansen, J. D., Schneider, B. A., Olive, B. M., and Bates, J. J.,** Personal safety and foliage residue in an orchard spraying program using Azinophosmethyl and Captan, *Arch. Environ. Contam. Toxicol.*, 7, 63, 1978.
44. **Wolfe, H. R., Durham, W. F., and Armstrong, J. F.,** Exposure of workers to pesticides, *Arch. Environ. Health*, 14, 622, 1967.
45. **Batchelor, G. S. and Walker, K. C.,** Health hazards involved in the use of parathion in fruit orchards of North Central Washington, *Arch. Ind. Hyg. Occup. Med.*, 10, 522, 1954.
46. **Katsenovich, A. I. and Usmanova, I. Y.,** On the appearance of liver autoantibodies in persons in contact with pesticides, *Med. Zh. Uzb.*, 7, 6, 1970.
47. **Kotlarek-Haus, S., Dzierzkowa-Borodej, W., and Lawinska, B.,** Autoimmune hemolytic anemia after handling insecticides and herbicides, with simultaneous detection of the Australia antigen (Au 1) in the serum, *Folia Haematol. (Leipzig)*, 95, 249, 1971.
48. **Brusilovskii, S. S., Vieveskii, N. A., Zinchenko, D. V., and Fialkovskii, A. M.,** Clinical and experimental study of the component during action of chemical substances, *Immunologiya*, 6, 72, 1973.
49. **Allazov, S.,** Autoantibodies toward tissue of the thyroid gland after bone fracture and during chronic butiphos poisoning, *Med. Zh. Uzb.*, 12, 20, 1973.
50. **Aripdzhanov, T. M.,** Effect of pesticides anthio and milbex on the immunologic reactivity and certain autoimmune processes of the body, *Gig. Sanit.*, 38, 39, 1973.
51. **Omirov, P. Y. and Talan, K. A.,** Rabbit autoimmunization under conditions of chronic poisoning with hexachlordane (BHC) and methyl mercaptophos, *Med. Zh. Uz.*, 7, 11, 1970.
52. **Nikolaev, A. I., Subkhankulova, F. B., and Geller, I. S.,** Immune reactions of poisoning with toxic chemicals: methylmercaptophos, phosphamide, aldrin, and monuron, *Russ. Pharmacol. Toxicol.*, 33, 322, 1970.
53. **Dodson, V. N., Mitchell, I., Friberg, R., and Ketchum, D.,** The role of autoimmunity in carbon tetrachloride intoxication: I. Influence of route of administration, *Toxicol. Appl. Pharmacol.*, 7, 482, 1965.
54. **Wassermann, M., Wassermann, D., Kedar, E., and Djavaherian, M.,** Effects of dieldrin and gamma BHC on serum proteins and PBI, *Bull. Environ. Contam. Toxicol.*, 8, 177, 1972.
55. **Wassermann, M., Kedar, E., Djavaherian, M., Cucos, S., and Ventura, S.,** Effect of organochlorine compounds on serum proteins, *Bull. Environ. Contam. Toxicol*, 10, 42, 1973.
56. **Friend, M. and Trainer, D. O.,** Experimental dieldrin-duck hepatitis virus interaction studies, *J. Wildl. Manage.*, 38, 896, 1974.
57. **Trepanier, G., Marchessault, F., Bansal, J., and Chagnon, A.,** Cytological effects of insecticides on a human lymphoblastoid cell line, *In Vitro*, 13, 201, 1977.
58. **Loose, L. D., Pittman, K. A., Benitz, K., and Silkworth, J. B.,** PCB and HCB induced immunosuppression in mice, *Toxicol. Appl. Pharmacol.*, 41, 201, 1977.
59. **Wassermann, M., Wassermann, D., Gershon, Z., and Zellermayer, L.,** Effects of organochlorine insecticides on body defense systems, *Ann. N.Y. Acad. Sci.*, 160, 393, 1969.

60. **Wassermann, M., Wassermann, D., Kedar, E., and Djavaherian, M.,** Immunological and detoxication interaction in p,p-DDT fed rabbits, *Bull. Environ. Contam. Toxicol.*, 6, 426, 1971.
61. **Wassermann, M. and Wassermann, D.,** Effects of organochlorine insecticides on homeostatic and immunologic processes, *Fate of Pesticides in the Environment,* Gordon and Breach, London, 1972, p 521.
62. **Olefir, A. I.** A study of the effect of chemical substances on the formation of acquired immunity, *Vrach. Delo,* 10, 125, 1971.
63. **Radhakrishnan, C. V., Thompson, N. P., and Forester, D. J.,** Susceptibility of chickens fed p,p-DDT to histomoniasis, *Bull. Environ, Contam. Toxicol.*, 8, 147, 1972.
64. **Perelygin, V. M., Shpirt, M. B., Aripov, O. A., and Ershova, V. I.,** Effects of some pesticides on immunological reactivity, *Gig. Sanit.*, 36, 29, 1971.
65. **Glick, B.,** Antibody-mediated immunity in the presence of mirex and DDT, Poultry Sci., 53, 1476, 1974.
66. **Subba Rao, D. S. V. and Glick, B.,** Pesticide effects on immune responses and metabolic activity of chicken lymphocytes, *Proc. Soc. Exp. Biol. Med.*, 154, 27, 1977.
67. **Ziprin, R. L. and Fowler, S. R.,** Rosette-forming ability of alveolar macrophages from rat lung: inhibition by hexachlorobenzene, *Toxicol. Appl. Pharmacol.*, 39, 105, 1977.
68. **Loose, L. B., Silkworth, J. B., and Coulston, F.,** Impaired host defence in mice fed Aroclor 1242 or hexachlorobenzene for six weeks, *Toxicol. Appl. Pharmacol.*, 41, 203, 1977.
69. **Rodica, G. and Stefania, M.,** [Effects of some insecticides on the bursa of Fabricius in chicks], *Arch. Exp. Veterinaermed.*, 27, 723, 1973.
70. **Park, B. H. and Lee, T. P.,** Effects of pesticides on human leukocyte function, in *Proceeding of the 4th FDA Science Symposium,* Asher, I. M., Ed., Annapolis, Md. 1978, 273.
71. **Crocker, J. F. S., Ozere, R. L., Safe, S. H., Digout, S. C., Rozee, K. R., and Hutzinger, O.,** Lethal interaction of ubiquitous insecticide carriers with virus, *Science,* 192, 1351, 1976.
72. **Koller, L. D., Exon, J. H., and Roan, J. G.,** Immunological surveillance and toxicity in mice exposed to the organophosphate pesticide, leptophos, *Environ. Res.*, 12, 238, 1976.
73. **Woodin, A. M. and Harris, A.,** The inhibition of locomotion of the polymorphonuclear leucocytes by organophosphorus compounds, *Exp. Cell Res.*, 77, 41, 1973.
74. **Nikolaev, A. I., Ponomareva, L. A., Geller, I. S., Rozgon, M. I., and Garipova, F. S.,** Immunodepressive action of some poisonous chemicals, *Farmakol. Toksikol. (Moscow),* 35, 352, 1972.
75. **Desi, T. F., Varga, G., and Judit, C. G.,** Immune suppressive effect of chlorinated hydrocarbon and organic phosphate pesticide administration, *Egeszsegtudomany,* 20, 358, 1976.
76. **Lis, T. and Mierzejewski, J.,** [Effect of foschlor and teration on the activity of guinea pig complement], *Med. Dosw. Mikrobiol.*, 25, 345, 1973.
77. **Fan, A., Street, J. C., and Nelson, R. M.,** Immunesuppression in mice administered methyl parathion and carbofuran by diet, *Toxicol. Appl. Pharmacol.*, 45, 235, 1978.
78. **Shtenberg, A. I. and Dzhunusova, R. M.,** Depression of immunobiological reaction of an animal under the influence of certain organophosphoric pesticides, *Bull. Exp. Biol. Med. (Russ.),* 33, 86, 1968.
79. **Olefir, A. I.,** Effect of chronic carbamate pesticide poisoning on immunologic responses and infection resistance, *Vrach. Delo,* 8, 137, 1973.
80. **Olefir, A. I., Effect of acute carbamate pesticide poisoning on immunologic responses,** *Vrach. Delo,* 4, 138, 1973.
81. **Bolkhovitianova, V. M. and Kogan, R. F.,** The effect of sevin on the immunobiological reactivity of the organism, *Faktory Vneshn. Sredy Ikh Znach. Zdorov ya Naseleniya,* 1, 129, 1969.
82. **Bolkhovitianova, V. M. and Aleksevich, I. A.,** The effect of the pesticide sevin on the formation of antitoxic immunity in experimental animals, *Vrach. Delo,* 8, 116, 1968.
83. **Shtenberg, A. I., Ashmenskas, Y. I., and Kusevitskiy, I. A.,** Immunobiological reactivity changes under the influence of some pesticides belonging to the group of carbamate and dithiocarbamate compounds, *Vopr. Pitan.*, 31, 58, 1972.
84. **Dinoeva, S. K.,** Dynamics of changes in the immune structure of lymphatic follicles of the spleen following pesticide poisoning, *Gig. Sanit.*, 3, 85, 1974.
85. **Aripdzhanov, T. M.,** Experimental study of the effects of anthio and milbex on immunologic reactivity and certain autoimmune processes of the body, *Gig. Sanit.*, 38, 101, 1973.
86. **Styles, J. A.,** Studies on the effects of paraquat and diquat on cells in culture. Viability of macrophages and fibroblasts incubated with paraquat and diquat, *Br. J. Exp. Pathol.*, 55, 71, 1974.
87. **Verschuuren, H. G., Ruitenberg, E. J., Peetoom, F., Helleman, P. W., and van Esch, G. F.,** Influence of triphenyltin acetate on lymphatic tissue and immune responses in guinea pigs, *Toxicol. Appl. Pharmacol.*, 16, 400, 1970.
88. **Street, J. C. and Sharma, R. P.,** Alteration of induced cellular and humoral immune responses by pesticides and chemicals of environmental concern: Quantitative studies of immunosuppression by DDT, Aroclor 1254, carbaryl, carbofuran, and methyl parathion, *Toxicol. Appl. Pharmacol.*, 32, 587, 1975.

89. **Gavat, V., Alexa, L., and Melinte, C.,** Studies on immunobiologic reactivity as an indicator for evaluating disturbances in the balance between the organism and the environment, *Igiena,* 25, 307, 1976.
90. **Wiltrout, R. W., Ercegovich, C. D., and Ceglowski, W. S.,** Humoral immunity in mice following administration of selected pesticides, *Bull. Environ. Contam. Toxicol.,* 20, 423, 1978.
91. **Sharma, R. P. and Street, J. C.,** unpublished data.
92. **Fan, A.,** Effects of pesticides on immune competency: Influence of methyl Parathion and Carbofuran on Immunologic Responses to *Salmonella typhimurium* infection, Ph.D. dissertation, Utah State University, Logan, 1980.
93. **Adkinson, N. F., Jr.,** Environmental influences on the immune system and allergic reactions, *Environmental Health Persp.,* 20, 97, 1977.

Chapter 7

IMMUNOLOGIC EFFECTS OF METALS

L. D. Koller and J. G. Vos

TABLE OF CONTENTS

INTRODUCTION

Many metals such as lead, cadmium, arsenic, and mercury are toxic to animals and humans, often producing disease or death after acute or chronic exposure. Adverse effects resulting from long-term subclinical levels of exposure, comparable to occupational or environmental conditions, are less well known. However, recent experiments have shown that chronic low-level exposure to certain metals may induce subtle changes within a host, including alteration of the immune response. This chapter will be concerned primarily with those metals which are considered to be environmental pollutants and therefore are potential hazards to public health. Metals such as chromium, platinum, gold, copper, manganese, cobalt, thorium, zinc, and iron will be discussed only briefly as will the production of contact hypersensitivity by metals since they are described elsewhere.[1]

In 1966, it was reported[2] that a single intravenous injection of lead acetate increased the sensitivity of rats to endotoxins of various Gram-negative bacteria about 100,000 times above normal. This was followed by similar studies in mice[3] and chickens[4] demonstrating that lead acetate enhanced responsiveness to bacterial endotoxins. Cadmium acetate induced similar changes in rats exposed to *Salmonella enteriditis* endotoxin.[5] It was apparent from these studies that at least two metals, lead and cadmium, greatly increased the susceptibility of animals to endotoxins.

Later, in 1971, it was demonstrated that mice treated with subclinical doses of lead nitrate showed greater susceptibility to challenge with *S. typhimurium* than controls which did not receive lead.[6] Other studies have described similar results using arsenicals,[7] cobalt sulfate,[8] cadmium,[9] and methylmercury.[10] Therefore it has been well established that certain metals render hosts more susceptible to infectious disease.

II. STUDIES WITH LEAD AND CADMIUM

The majority of the studies with lead and cadmium dealt with increased susceptibility to infection with Gram-negative bacteria that contain endotoxin. This is probably the result of the observation of Selye and co-workers that lead greatly increases the susceptibility of rats to bacterial endotoxin. Mortality and organ changes normally produced by the intravenous injection of 100 μg of *Escherichia coli* endotoxin were essentially the same as those obtained by use of 1 ng in rats intravenously injected with 5 mg lead acetate per 100 g body weight, which is a normally well tolerated dose of lead.[1] In the same report, the increased vulnerability of lead treated rats to bacterial infection was first demonstrated by the injection of viable and killed fecal flora. The sensitizing effect of lead for *E. coli* endotoxin was greatest when the two agents were given simultaneously; considerable sensitization was still detectable when endotoxin was injected up to 1 hr before or 7 hr after sensitization with lead. Cook et al.[9] reported that an acute dose of lead acetate enhanced the susceptibility of rats to intravenous challenge with *E. coli* by approximate 1000-fold. Equivalent vulnerability was found with killed *E. coli*. An equal dose of the Gram-positive *Staphylococcus epidermidis* failed to produce mortality, although a ten times higher dose did give more deaths than observed in the nonlead treated animals. The synthetic glucocorticoid, methylprednisolone, prevented lethality induced by *E. coli* in lead treated rats. These data indicate that lead treatment results in a profound increase in the susceptibility to bacterial endotoxin as has been shown in several other studies.[11]

In the mouse, lead treatment resulted in decreased resistance to Gram-negative bacteria. Mice were given daily intraperitoneal injections with different doses of lead nitrate. During the 30 day period of exposure, no signs of toxicity were observed. Upon challenge with low doses of *Salmonella typhimurium,* the mortality in the lead treated mice was significantly higher than in the controls.[6] According to these authors, a logical explanation would be that lead interferes with a resistance mechanism in the mice, thereby permitting inhibited bacterial growth, resulting in the production of lethal quantities of endotoxin.

Lead also decreased the resistance to viral infections. Gainer[12] reported that splenomegaly (with high titers of virus) could be induced in lead treated mice after injection with Rauscher leukemia virus. Lead also increased the mortality in mice that were infected with encephalomyocarditis virus or pseudorabies virus. Lead did depress the antiviral activity of the interferon inducer poly I/poly C, but did not influence the antiviral activity of interferon either in vivo or in vitro. Thus lead seems to aggravate viral disease, most likely through reduced interferon synthesis but not via inhibition of interferon action.[13] Depressed interferon response is reported by Vengris and Mare[14] in chickens that were given a toxic dose of lead acetate P.O., but no effect was seen in animals receiving a subclinical level. In addition, antibody titers to Newcastle disease virus were not depressed by lead treatment.

The effect of lead on the antibody response in rabbits was studied by Koller.[15] The primary and secondary response to pseudorabies virus in rabbits after treatment with 2500 ppm lead acetate in their drinking water for 10 weeks was severely depressed. However, weight gain of the animals was severely depressed, thus it is questionable whether the animals received a subclinical dose of the compound. Mice receiving a single oral or intraperitoneal dose of 4 mg of lead acetate, a dose that did not produce histopathological alterations in kidney and liver, had a significantly increased number of IgM plaque forming cells to Sheep Red Blood Cells (SRBC). The secondary (IgG) antibody response (as measured with the indirect plaque technique) was significantly reduced in mice exposed orally and particularly in those inoculated intraperitoneally with lead.[16] Exposure of mice to 1375, 137.5, or 13.75 ppm lead acetate in the drinking water did result in each dose group in a significantly decreased number of antibody forming cells to SRBC (IgM and particularly IgG); histopathological examination of the kidney disclosed a dose-related necrosis of tubular epithelial cells in the cortex.[17] In an extensive study of Trejo et al.[18] with adult rats given a single intravenous injection of 5 mg lead acetate, no effect was found on the primary and secondary antibody response to SRBC. A similar treatment with lead did, however, result in a significantly depressed intravascular clearance of colloidal carbon starting at 6 hr after lead treatment, thus contrasting with the enhanced susceptibility to endotoxin which occurs when lead and endotoxin are administered simultaneously. Also, the intravascular removal of ^{131}I-triolein-labeled lipid emulsion was depressed. Associated with the impaired vascular clearance, there was a marked reduction in the hepatic phagocytosis but some increase in the uptake of spleen and lung. In addition, altered liver function tests indicated the presence of acute hepatic injury. The endotoxin detoxifying ability of liver and spleen homogenates from lead-treated rats was significantly lower when compared with homogenates of controls. Depressed clearance of colloidal carbon that already was apparent 15 min after treatment with lead, was observed by Filkins and Buchanan,[19] but in contrast, no differences were noted in the vascular clearance of endotoxin in lead treated rats. Similar observations were made in lead acetate-treated mice.[20]

In addition to lead, cadmium strongly increases the susceptibility of rats to *E. coli* infection, and equivalent vulnerability was found of cadmium treated rats to killed *E. coli*[9]. Although there is a striking similarity in the susceptibility to endotoxin of rats treated with lead or cadmium, a difference is manifested by the inability of methylprednisolone to modify mortality in cadmium-endotoxin-induced shock, as opposed to its protective effect in lead-endotoxin shock.[11]

Koller[15] found reduced primary and secondary antibody responses to pseudorabies virus in rabbits after 10 week exposure to 300 ppm cadmium chloride in their drinking water, but a moderate decrease in weight gain was observed in the treated animals when compared with the controls. Mice exposed to 3 or 300 ppm cadmium chloride in the drinking water for 10 weeks, and inoculated with SRBC during cadmium exposure or 1, 7, 14, or 42 days after exposure had a decreased number of antibody forming cells (IgM and particularly IgG). In both treatment groups, there was damage of the kidneys, especially in the 300 ppm group.[21] Seemingly conflicting results of the effect of cadmium on the humoral immune response are reported by Jones et al.[22] Rats that received subcutaneous injections of 0.6 mg cadmium chloride per kg body weight, 5 days/week, had significantly increased primary and secondary antibody responses to human gamma globulin when injections of cadmium started 2 weeks before the first antigen injection. On the contrary, cadmium doses initiated 1 week before the first antigen injection delayed and suppressed the primary and secondary antibody responses, respectively. Cadmium injections initiated two days after the second antigen injection did result in a depression of the secondary antibody response. Different responses after cadmium exposure were also reported by Koller et al.[16] The primary and secondary antibody response to SRBC (as determined by the number of plaque forming cells) were increased when mice received a single intraperitoneal injection, whereas depressed antibody responses were found when the animals received a single oral dose of 0.15 mg cadmium chloride.

In conclusion, it is well established that both lead and cadmium greatly increase the susceptibility to endotoxin and to infection with endotoxin containing bacteria (Table 1), although the mechanisms of action of both compounds are probably not quite the same. Lead also induced impairment of hepatic macrophage activity, but since maximum impairment is present at a time when rats become less sensitive to endotoxin, it does not seem likely that alteration in phagocytic function is a primary factor in sensitivity to endotoxin.[11,18] As discussed by these authors, several factors, either alone or in combination, may elicit a cascade of reactions culminating in the death of the animal; factors such as impairment of the endotoxin detoxifying properties of macrophages (perhaps by inactivation of sulfhydryl containing enzymes necessary for endotoxin inactivation), or hepatic parenchymal cell dysfunction by lead-induced liver injury. Although less drastically, lead exposure also increases the vulnerability to several viral infections, most likely through reduced synthesis of interferon and not via inhibition of interferon action, as well as it increases the sensibility to infection with a Gram-positive microorganism. It does not seem likely that impaired humoral immunity plays a role in the increased susceptibility to infection with endotoxin containing bacteria and with viruses, although the effects of lead and cadmium on the immune response are difficult to assess. First, varying responses (enhancement, reduction, or no effect) seem to be at least partly, due to differences in route of administration, single dose vs. semichronic exposure, and time of antigenic stimulation. Next, an impaired humoral immune response was associated in some studies with reduced weight gain or histopathological lesions, which could indirectly be responsible for the reduced antibody synthesis. Thirdly, lead decreases the phagocytic clearance; thus a reduced immune response could be due to impaired antigen processing or presentation by macrophages. Finally, when there is an effect, it concerns in particular the IgG response, which is considered to be more thymus-dependent than the IgM response. Therefore, future studies should give attention to T-helper cells. In addition, the effect of lead and cadmium on the cell-mediated immunity needs investigation, since function studies that are reported up to now, concentrate on the humoral immunity.

Table 1
THE EFFECT OF IN VIVO LEAD OR CADMIUM EXPOSURE ON SUSCEPTIBILITY TO INFECTION AND ON VARIOUS IMMUNOLOGICAL PARAMETERS

Chemical	Species	Parameter	Effect[a]	Ref.
Lead acetate	Rat	Susceptibility fecal flora infection	+	2
Lead nitrate	Mouse	Susceptibility *Salmonella typhimurium* infection	+	6
Lead acetate	Rat	Susceptibility *E. coli* infection	++	9
		Susceptibility heat killed *E. coli*	++	9
		Susceptibility *E. coli* infection + methylprednisolone	−	9
		Susceptibility *Staphylococcus epidermidis* infection	+	9
	Mouse	Activation Rauscher leukemia virus	+	12
		Susceptibility encephalomyocarditis virus	+	13
		Susceptibility pseudorabies virus	+	13
		Depression interferon synthesis	+	13
		Interferon action	−	13
	Chicken	Depression interferon synthesis	−/+[b]	14
		Antibody response to Newcastle disease virus	−/−[b]	14
	Rabbit	Antibody response to pseudorabies virus	+/+[c]	15
	Mouse	IgM antibody response to SRBC	−/+[d]	16, 17
		IgG antibody response to SRBC	+/+[e]	16, 17
	Rat	Antibody response to SRBC	−/−[c]	18
		Carbon and triolein clearance by macrophages	+	18
		Carbon clearance by macrophages	+	19
	Mouse	Carbon clearance by macrophages	+	20
Cadmium acetate	Rat	Susceptibility *E. coli* infection	++	9
		Susceptibility heat killed *E. coli*	++	9
		Susceptibility *E. coli* infection + methylprednisolone	++	9
Cadmium chloride	Rabbit	Antibody response to pseudorabies virus	+/+[c]	15
	Mouse	Antibody response to SRBC	+/+[c]	21
	Rat	Antibody response to human gamma globulin	−/+[f]	22
	Mouse	Antibody response to SRBC	−/+[g]	16

[a] Denotes the increased susceptibility to infection and the suppressive effect on immunological parameters; + = slight to moderate, ++ = strong; − = no effect.

[b] Respectively subclinical and toxic levels.

[c] Respectively on the primary and secondary antibody response.

[d] Respectively increased antibody response with single dose exposure (orally or intraperitoneally) and decrease with semichronic exposure.

[e] Respectively single dose (orally or intraperitoneally) and semichronic exposure.

[f] Primary and secondary antibody response were respectively increased or decreased when cadmium injections were initiated two weeks or one week before the first antigen injection.

[g] Respectively increased primary and secondary antibody response after a single intraperitoneal injection and decrease after single oral exposure.

III. ARSENICALS

Gainer and Pry[23] studied the effect of arsenicals on viral infections in mice (Table 2). Four-week old mice were treated with the compounds in several ways: continuously in the drinking water (at a concentration of 0.002 *M*) 1 or 2 weeks before or 1 day after virus inoculation, and single or repeated subcutaneous injections of 3.13 or 6.25 mg sodium arsenite, 5.0 mg arsenic trioxide, or 25 mg *p*-arsanilic acid per kg body weight. With most arsenicals, virus-infected mice had two to ninefold higher rates of mortality than untreated controls. Susceptibility of mice to pseudorabies infection was increased by sodium arsenite, arsenic trioxide, and sodium arsenate; increased mortality did also occur in mice infected with encephalomyocarditis virus and exposed to sodium arsenite or 4-hydroxy-3-nitrobenzenearsonic acid, but not to *p*-arsanilic acid. Treatment with 4-hydroxy-3-nitrobenzenearsonic acid increased the susceptibility of mice to St. Louis encephalitis virus and to Western encephalitis virus when treatment started 1 day after virus inoculation. In contrast, exposure of mice to sodium arsenite did reduce the mortality after infection with Western encephalitis virus. Treatment with sodium arsenite and *p*-arsanilic acid did increase the frequency of splenomegaly and viral titer in spleen and plasma of mice infected with Rauscher leukemogenic virus. These data indicate that most arsenicals increase the susceptibility to viral infections. But, mice given arsenicals in the drinking water for 1 to 3 weeks before they were inoculated with viral material were retarded in growth, and a few mice died before viral inoculation. Thus, it can not be excluded that the increased mortality is indirectly due to a toxic action of the arsenicals, since experiments with noninoculated virus controls treated with the different arsenicals were not included.

A possible explanation for the increase of viral deaths in mice by arsenicals is presented in a subsequent study of Gainer;[24] high concentrations of arsenicals inhibited both the synthesis and the action of interferon, whereas low concentrations of arsenicals increased the antiviral activity of low levels of interferon. The beneficial growth-promoting effects of arsenicals as feed additives through reduction in disease may be in part through this increased interferon activity. Gainer and Pry[23] considered it unlikely that a reduced antibody formation accounts for the enhancement of viral disease by arsenicals, since essentially the same patterns were noted in tissue culture. But it was shown more than 5 decades ago, that low concentrations of arsphenamine increased antibody production, whereas high concentrations inhibited it[25] Thus, one can argue that relatively high concentrations of arsenicals increase the susceptibility to viral disease, not only through an effect on interferon, but also by impairment of the immune response. This is clearly an area for future research.

IV. MERCURY

Koller[10] and Koller et al.[26] studied the effect of methylmercury chloride on viral infection. Mice were fed this compound at levels of 0, 1, or 10 ppm for 84 days. The latter dose did not produce death, but necrosis of proximal convoluted tubules was present in the kidneys. Inoculation of a high dose of encephalomyocarditis virus at day 70 did increase the mortality in the 1 and 10 ppm group when compared with the controls, whereas a low dose of virus only produced an increased mortality rate at the 10 ppm level. In contrast, the response of methylmercury treated mice to Rauscher leukemia virus did not significantly differ from the respective control animals. Ohi and co-authors[27] studied the effect of methylmercury chloride on the primary and secondary antibody response to SRBC. In the first experiment mice were intubated orally with doses of 0, 0.34, or 3.4 mg/kg body weight for 5 consecutive days (the LD_{50} of

Table 2

THE EFFECT OF IN VIVO EXPOSURE OF MICE TO ARSENICALS ON SUSCEPTIBILITY TO VIRAL INFECTION

Chemical	Parameter	Effect[a]	Ref.
Sodium arsenite	Susceptibility to pseudorabies infection	+[b,c]	23
Arsenic trioxide	Susceptibility to pseudorabies infection	+[b]	23
Sodium arsenate	Susceptibility to pseudorabies infection	+[c]	23
Sodium arsenite	Susceptibility to encephalomyocarditis infection	+[b,c]	23
p-Arsanilic acid	Susceptibility to encephalomyocarditis infection	−[b]	23
4-Hydroxy-3-nitrobenzenearsonic acid	Susceptibility to encephalomyocarditis infection	+[c]	23
4-Hydroxy-3-nitrobenzenearsonic acid	Susceptibility to St. Louis encephalitis infection	+[c,d]	23
4-Hydroxy-3-nitrobenzenearsonic acid	Susceptibility to Western encephalitis infection	−[c]/+[d]	23
Sodium arsenite	Susceptibility to Western encephalitis infection	−[e]	23
Sodium arsenite	Susceptibility to Rauscher leukemogenic infection	+[f]	23
p-Arsanilic acid	Susceptibility to Rauscher leukemogenic infection	+[f]	23

[a] Denotes the effect: + = slight to moderate; − = no effect.
[b] Subcutaneous injection of chemical at time of virus inoculation.
[c] Treatment in the drinking water 1 or 2 weeks before virus inoculation.
[d] Treatment in the drinking water 1 day after virus inoculation.
[e] Reduced mortality by subcutaneous injection of chemical at time of virus inoculation.
[f] Subcutaneous injection of chemical at time of virus inoculation and continuing 3 times each week for 8 weeks.

methylmercury chloride being 34 mg/kg). On day 6 and 10 the animals were inoculated with SRBC. Primary and secondary antibody responses were determined respectively by the direct or indirect plaque forming cell response. In a second experiment, groups of female mice were given diets containing 0, 0.5 or 5 ppm methylmercury at the time of mating. The exposure of the offspring continued until 6 weeks after weaning. In a third experiment, 6 weeks old mice received diets containing 0, 0.5, or 5 ppm methylmercury for 12 weeks. The primary immune response was suppressed and delayed in experiment 1 (mice receiving 3.4 mg methylmercury/kg for 5 days), but the secondary response was not suppressed. Mice receiving 5 ppm in the diet had primary (experiments 2 and 3) and secondary (experiment 2) plaque forming cell responses that tended to be depressed, but at this dose level a slight reduction in body weight was noted towards the end of both experiments. In all three experiments no effect was found on weight and histology of thymus and spleen. Koller[15] found reduced primary and secondary antibody responses to pseudorabies virus in rabbits after 10 week exposure to 10 ppm mercuric chloride in the drinking water, but a slight decrease in weight gain was observed in the mercury group when compared with the control animals. The immunologic effects of mercury and selected other metals are summarized in Table 3.

Table 3

THE EFFECT OF IN VIVO EXPOSURE TO SELECTED METALS ON SUSCEPTIBILITY TO INFECTION AND ON VARIOUS IMMUNOLOGICAL PARAMETERS

Chemical	Species	Parameter	Effect[a]	Ref.
Methylmercury chloride	Mouse	Susceptibility to encephalomyocarditis virus	+	10
		Activation Rauscher leukemia virus	—	10
		Antibody response to SRBC	+/+[b]	26
Mercury chloride	Rabbit	Antibody response to pseudorabies virus	+/+[c]	15
Cobalt sulfate	Mouse	Susceptibility to encephalomyocarditis virus	+	27
		Activation Rauscher leukemia virus	+	12
Nickel acetate	Rat	Antibody response T-1 phage	+	28
Disodium chromate	Rat	Antibody response to T-1 phage	+	28

[a] Denotes the increased susceptibility to infection and the suppressive effect on immunological parameters: + = slight to moderate; ++ = strong; — = no effect.

[b] Respectively suppression and delay of primary antibody response after short-term treatment with a relatively large amount, and marginal reduction of primary and secondary response after subchronic feeding of low levels.

[c] Respectively on the primary and secondary antibody response.

V. OTHER METALS

The effect of cobalt sulfate on viral infections was studied by Gainer.[12,28] Mice receiving 47 ppm cobalt sulfate in their drinking water for 75 days had a twofold higher mortality when exposed to encephalomyocarditis virus than did nontreated viral controls.[28] Treatment of the mice with cobalt sulfate did not reduce weight gain or peripheral lymphocyte count, and did not result in pathological lesions. In cell culture experiments, cobalt sulfate did inhibit interferon activity which according to the author may be a principal factor in explaining the in vivo actions of cobalt sulfate on encephalomyocarditis virus. A similar mechanism may be responsible for the activation of Rauscher leukemia virus (splenomegaly with high titers of virus) in mice treated with 0.01 *M* cobalt sulfate in the drinking water.

Figoni and Treagan[29] studied the effect of nickel and chromium on the humoral immunity. Rats were given subcutaneous injections of 10.7 mg nickel acetate of 13.3 mg disodium chromate per kg body weight, every other day. Treatment started between 2 weeks before and 12 days after the first immunization. Animals received 3 antigen injections, at 10 day intervals, of *E. coli* bacteriophage T-1. Antibody titers, determined by the phage neutralization test, were depressed, particularly when treatment with the metals started early. However, the rats were given a dose that represent one third of the LD_{50} and no further data are presented. Thus it is difficult to evaluate the significance of the observed suppression of the humoral immunity.

There has been considerable interest in nickel toxicity since the metal was implicated as a possible etiology for "Legionnaires Disease". Even though nickel had not caused death in the Legionnaires, nickel concentrations were elevated in lung tissues nine times that of controls.[30] Koller,[31] found that large doses of nickel chloride did not alter infectivity of encephalomyocarditis virus in mice. However, it has been reported that nickel acetate depressed circulating antibody titers[32] to T-1 phage as well as inhibited the interferon response of metal-treated cells.[33] Further investigations need to be conducted to elucidate the function of nickel on the immune response.

Administration of other metals such as cobalt,[34] chromium,[32] and platinum[35] has been reported to suppress the immune system. Diets deficient in copper[36,37,38], zinc,[36] iron,[36,39] manganese,[37] or magnesium,[40] have also resulted in a diminished immune response. The studies involving tin (particularly organotin) compounds will be described in Chapter 10 of this volume.

Not all metals suppress the immune system. Selenium has been shown to enhance the immune response by increasing the number of antibody forming cells.[41] The response was greatest when selenium was administered prior to or simultaneously with the antigen. Other metals such as copper, manganese, and cobalt have been reported by some investigators to enhance[42-44] the immune response while others observed suppression[34-37] of the immune system by the same. It is obvious from these studies that many metals influence the immune system. Those which interfere with normal function of the immune response are of considerable concern to public health.

VI. EFFECTS OF METALS ON IMMUNOCOMPETENT CELL POPULATIONS

Since it has been confirmed that numerous metals, often at subclinical doses, inhibit the immune response, their action on lymphocytes, plasma cells, accessory cells or a combination thereof must be examined. Antibody responses to many antigens require cooperation between at least two types of lymphocytes for optimal expression. One cell type is thymus-derived (T cells). T cells may amplify, help or suppress B cells as well as function as cytotoxic cells. T cells do not produce antibody. The other cell type is bone marrow-derived (B cells) and matures independently of thymic influence. B cells differentiate into antibody-producing cells and are often influenced by T cells. A third cell type is the macrophage which has an important role as an accessory cell by cooperating with T cells in aiding the response of B cells to antigens.

Experiments recently conducted[31] have examined the effect of lead and cadmium on B cells. After 10 weeks of exposure to the metals, spleens were collected and examined for the ability of B cells to form rosettes using an erythrocyte-antibody-complement (EAC) assay.[38] Fewer EAC rosettes were formed by splenic B lymphocytes from mice exposed to lead or cadmium than by B cells from control animals. The direct effect of these compounds on B cells could account in part for their suppression of the humoral immune response (Table 4).

It has also been determined that both lead and cadmium activated macrophages instead of suppressing their activity.[45] These two metals stimulated phagocytosis (Table 5) and increased acid phosphatase levels in macrophages. Since lead and cadmium primarily suppress the secondary immune response, the moderately reduced primary response may be due to direct action of these compounds on B cells as discussed above.[38] The increased ability of macrophages to phagocytize and contribute to immunogenicity of the antigen may not be great enough to compensate for this inhibition. Accordingly, macrophages influence the primary, but not the secondary, immune response and therefore would not interfere with the markedly suppressed secondary response.

Other studies[46,47] disclosed that a single intravenous injection of lead acetate impaired Kupffer cell phagocytosis. Several factors must be considered in these studies. First, it has been reported[16] that single doses of lead and cadmium produce different results than do prolonged exposures. Secondly, route of administration influences the type of immune response. Intravenous challenge would be conducive to an intense response compared to

Table 4
METALS THAT ALTER HUMORAL ANTIBODY TITERS

Metal	Antigen	Antibody Titer	
		Increased	Decreased
Lead	Pseudorabies virus		X
Cadmium	Pseudorabies virus		X
Mercury	Pseudorabies virus		X
Methylmercury	Influenza virus		X
Nickel	T-1 phage		X
Cobalt	horse serum		X
Chromium	T-1 phage		X
Platinum	Sheep Red Blood Cells (SRBC)		X
Selenium	SRBC	X	
Copper	SRBC	X	
Manganese	SRBC	X	

Table 5
METALS THAT ALTER PHAGOCYTOTIC ACTIVITY OF MACROPHAGES

Metal	Material Phagocytized	Phagocytosis	
		Increased	Decreased
Lead	SRBC	X	
Cadmium	SRBC	X	
Lead	Colloidal carbon		X
Nickel	latex spheres		X
Zinc	*Staphylococcus albus*		X

oral exposure. Finally, other factors such as opsonins are involved in in vivo studies. Lead and cadmium may inhibit opsonins or other soluble factors (alpha-2-globulin, etc.) that could perhaps oppose the stimulatory effect observed in the in vitro experiments. Two other metals, nickel[48] and zinc,[49] have also been shown to inhibit the phagocytic ability of macrophages. The alteration of phagocytosis by alveolar macrophages as influenced by several trace metals has been described.[48]

Preliminary data[31] indicated that lead and cadmium also inhibit lymphocyte transformation of T cells stimulated by Con A. Therefore, it is apparent that certain metals affect T cells by inhibiting cell division. Such inhibition of T cells suggests impairment of cell mediated immunity. Gaworski and Sharma[50] have described the inhibition of PHA and PWM induced mitogenesis in murine splenic cells after in vivo exposure to lead, cadmium, and mercury. Zinc caused a stimulation of such lymphocyte proliferation when mice were exposed to this metal. Both lead and zinc increased the response of lymphocytes to blastogenic agents when the metals were added in vitro, while the effect of cadmium and mercury was inhibitory.

Interferons have a marked inhibitory effect on antibody response, and several types of interferon can be produced by mammalian cells.[51] Virus-induced interferon is produced in lymphoid or nonlymphoid cells following stimulation by virus or double-stranded RNA. Mitogen-induced interferon is produced by lymphoid cells following stimulation by T lymphocyte mitogens. Antigen-induced interferon is produced in antigen-primed lymphoid cells upon second exposure to the specific antigen. Interferon could perhaps be altered by metals and thus contribute to the increased mortality rate in virus-inoculated animals since differences in sensitivity to interferon vary considerably among viruses. Cobalt sulfate,[8] sodium arsenite,[24] and nickel acetate,[33] have been shown to inhibit the action of interferon while other metals such as cadmium, iron and chromium may not affect interferon production.

VII. CONCLUSION

It has been well established that certain metals render hosts more susceptible to infectious disease. The mechanism of this synergism is related, at least in part, to the immunosuppressive properties of the metals. Therefore, it is apparent that such metals are indirectly detrimental to health, and exposure to these should be kept to a minimum.

REFERENCES

1. **Treagan, L.,** Metals and the immune response; A review, *Res. Comm. Chem. Path. Pharmacol.,* 12, 189, 1975.
2. **Selye, H., Tuchweber, B., and Bertok, L.,** Effect of lead acetate on the susceptibility of rats to bacterial endotoxins, *J. Bact.,* 91, 884, 1966.
3. **Rippe, D. F. and Berry, L. J.,** Metabolic manifestations of lead acetate sensitization to endotoxin in mice, *J. Reticuloendothel. Soc.,* 13, 527, 1973.
4. **Truscott, R. B.,** Endotoxin studies in chicks: effect of lead acetate, *Can. J. Comp. Med.,* 34, 134, 1970.
5. **Cook, J. A., Marconi, E. A., and DiLuzio, N. R.,** Lead, cadmium, endotoxin interaction: effect on mortality and hepatic function, *Toxicol. Appl. Pharmacol.,* 28, 292, 1974.
6. **Hemphill, F. E., Kaeberle, M. L., and Buck, W. B.,** Lead suppression of mouse resistance to *Salmonella typhimurium, Science,* 172, 1031, 1971.
7. **Gainer, J. H. and Pry, T. W.,** Effects of arsenicals on viral infections in mice, *Am. J. Vet. Res.,* 33, 2299, 1972.
8. **Gainer, J. H.,** Increased mortality in encephalomyocarditis virus-infected mice consuming cobalt sulfate: tissue concentrations of cobalt, *Am. J. Vet. Res.,* 33, 2067, 1972.
9. **Cook, J. A., Hoffman, E. O., and DiLuzio, N. R.,** Influence of lead and cadmium on the susceptibility of rats to bacterial challenge, *Proc. Soc. Exp. Biol. Med.,* 150, 741, 1975.
10. **Koller, L. D.,** Methylmercury: effect on oncogenic and nononcogenic viruses in mice, *Am. J. Vet. Res.,* 36, 1501, 1975.
11. **Cook, J. A., DiLuzio, N. R., and Hoffmann, E. O.,** Factors modifying susceptibility to bacterial endotoxin: the effect of lead and cadmium, *CRC Crit. Rev. Toxicol.,* 3, 201, 1975.
12. **Gainer, J. H.,** Activation of the Rauscher leukemia virus by metals, *J. Natl. Cancer Inst.,* 51, 609, 1973.
13. **Gainer, J. H.,** Lead aggravates viral disease and represses the antiviral activity of interferon inducers, *Environ. Health Perspect.,* 7, 113, 1974.
14. **Vengris, V. E. and Mare, C. J.,** Lead poisoning in chickens and the effect of lead on interferon and antibody production, *Can. J. Comp. Med.,* 38, 328, 1974.
15. **Koller, L. D.,** Immunosuppression produced by lead, cadmium and mercury, *Am. J. Vet. Res.,* 34, 1457, 1973.
16. **Koller, L. D., Exon, J. H., and Roan, J. G.,** Humoral antibody response in mice after single dose exposure to lead or cadmium, *Proc. Soc, Exp. Biol. Med.,* 151, 339, 1976.
17. **Koller, L. D. and Kovacic, S.,** Decreased antibody formation in mice exposed to lead, *Nature (London),* 250, 148, 1974.
18. **Trejo, R. A., DiLuzio, N. R., and Hoffmann, E. O.,** Reticuloendothelial and hepatic functional alterations following lead acetate administration, *Exp. Mol. Pathol.,* 17, 145, 1972.
19. **Filkins, J. P. and Buchanan, B. J.,** Effects of lead acetate on sensitivity to shock, intravascular carbon and endotoxin clearances and hepatic endo-toxin detoxification, *Proc. Soc. Exp. Biol. Med.,* 142, 471, 1973.
20. **Seyberth, H. W., Schmidt-Gayk, H., and Hackental, E.,** Toxicity, clearance and distribution of endotoxin in mice as influenced by actinomycin D, cycloheximide, α-amanitin and lead acetate, *Toxicon,* 10, 491, 1972.

21. **Koller, L. D., Exon, J. H., and Roan, J. G.,** Antibody suppression by cadmium, *Arch. Environ. Health*, 30, 598, 1975.
22. **Jones, R. H., Williams, R. L., and Jones, A. M.,** Effects of heavy metal on the immune response. Preliminary findings for cadmium in rats, *Proc. Soc. Exp. Biol. Med.*, 137, 1231, 1971.
23. **Gainer, J. H. and Pry, T. W.,** Effects of arsenicals on viral infections in mice, *Am. J. Vet. Res.*, 33, 2299, 1972.
24. **Gainer, J. H.,** Effects of arsenicals on interferon formation and action, *Am. J. Vet. Res.*, 33, 2579, 1972.
25. **Toyama, I. and Kolmer, J. A.,** The influence of arsphenamine and mercuric chloride upon complement and antibody production, *J. Immunol.*, 3, 301, 1918.
26. **Koller, L. D., Exon, J. H., and Arbogast, B.,** Methylmercury: effect on serum enzymes and humoral antibody, *J. Toxicol. Environ. Health*, 2, 1115, 1977.
27. **Ohi, G., Fukuda, M., Seto, H., and Yagyu, H.,** Effect of methylmercury on humoral immune responses in mice under conditions simulated to practical situations, *Bull. Environ. Contam. Toxicol.*, 15, 175, 1976.
28. **Gainer, J. H.,** Increased mortality in encephalomyocarditis virus-infected mice consuming cobalt sulfate: tissue concentrations of cobalt, *Am. J. Vet. Res.*, 33, 2067, 1972.
29. **Figoni, R. and Treagan, L.,** Inhibition effect of nickel and chromium upon antibody response of rats to immunization with T-1 phage, *Res. Commun. Chem. Path. Pharmacol.*, 11, 335, 1975.
30. **Chen, J. R., Francisco, R. B., and Miller, T. E.,** Legionnaires' Disease: nickel levels, *Science*, 196, 906, 1977.
31. **Koller, L. D.,** unpublished. *Private communication.*
32. **Figoni, R. and Treagan, L.,** Inhibition effect on nickel and chromium upon antibody response of rats to immunization with T-1 phage, *Res. Comm. Chem. Path. Pharmacol.*, 11, 335, 1975.
33. **Tregan, L. and Furst, A.,** Inhibition of interferon synthesis in mammalian cell cultures after nickel treatment, *Res. Comm. Chem. Path. Pharmacol.*, 1, 395, 1970.
34. **Derkach, V. V. and Burmakina, L. I.,** The influence of cobalt on precipitin formation and development of Arthus phenomenon, *Zh. Mikrobiol. Epidemiol. Immunobiol.*, 47, 59, 1970.
35. **Berenbaum, M. C.,** Immunosuppression by platinum diamines, *Br. J. Cancer*, 25, 208, 1971.
36. **Pakhomov, I. N.,** The significance of various micro-elements in the general immunologic reactivity of the animal body, *Zh. Mikrobiol. Epidemiol. Immunobiol.*, 47, 128, 1970.
37. **Kolomitseva, M. G., Voznesenskaia, F. M., and Isaeva, E. A.,** Immunobiologic reactivity of the animal organism with regard to various concentration of copper in its rations, *Zh. Mikrobiol. Epidemiol. Immunobiol.*, 46, 99, 1969.
38. **Koller, L. D. and Brauner, J. A.,** Decreased B cell response after exposure to lead and cadmium, *Toxicol. Appl. Pharmacol.* 42, 621, 1977.
39. **Nalder, B. N., Mahoney, A. W., Ramakrishnan, R., and Hendricks, D. G.,** Sensitivity of the immunological response to the nutritional status of rats, *J. Nutr.*, 102, 535, 1972.
40. **Elin, R. J.,** The effect of magnesium deficiency in mice on serum immunoglobulin concentrations and antibody plaque-forming cells, *Proc. Soc. Exp. Biol. Med.*, 148, 620, 1975.
41. **Spallholz, J. E., Martin, J. L., Gerlach, M. C., and Heinzerling, R. H.,** Injectable selenium: effect on the primary immune response of mice, *Proc. Soc. Exp. Biol. Med.*, 148, 37, 1975.
42. **Bazhora, I. I., Shtefen, E. E., and Timoshevski, I. V.,** The effect of microelements — copper, manganese and cobalt — on the antibody-forming function of lymphoid tissue, *Mikrobiol. Zh.*, 36, 771, 1974.
43. **Antonova, M. V., Pristupa, V. A., and Popov, V. P.,** Effect of small amounts of trace elements in the diet on immunological responses, *Gig. Sanit.*, 33, 39, 1968.
44. **Antonova, M. J.,** Effect of different amounts of manganese in the diet on immunological reactivity, *Vop. Pitan.*, 27, 36, 1968.
45. **Koller, L. D. and Roan, J. G.,** Effects of lead and cadmium on mouse peritoneal macrophages, *J. Reticuloendothel. Soc.*, 21, 7, 1977.
46. **Trejo, R. A., DiLuzio, N. R., Loose, L. D., and Hoffman, E.,** Reticuloendothelial and hepatic functional alterations following lead acetate administration, *Exp. Mol. Path.*, 17, 145, 1972.
47. **Filkins, J. P. and Buchanan, B. J.,** Effects of lead acetate on sensitivity to shock, intravascular carbon and endotoxin clearances, and hepatic endotoxin detoxification, *Proc. Soc. Exp. Biol. Med.*, 142, 471, 1973.
48. **Graham, J. A., Gardner, D. E., Waters, M. D., and Coffin, D. C.,** Effect of trace metals on phagocytosis by alveolar macrophages, *Infec. Immun.*, 11, 1278, 1975.
49. **Karl, L., Chrapi, M., and Zukoski, C. R.,** Effect of zinc on the viability and phagocytic capacity of peritoneal macrophages, *Proc. Soc. Exp. Biol. Med.*, 142, 1123, 1973.
50. **Gaworski, C. L. and Sharma, R. P.,** The effects of heavy metals on [^{3}H] thymidine uptake in lymphocytes, *Toxicol. Appl. Pharmacol.*, 46, 305, 1978.
51. **Johnson, H. M., Stanton, G. J., and Baron, S.,** Relative ability of mitogens to stimulate production of interferon by lymphoid cells and to induce suppression of the in vitro immune response, *Proc. Soc. Exp. Biol. Med.*, 154, 138, 1977.

Chapter 8

INDUSTRIAL COMPOUNDS AND MODIFICATION OF IMMUNE RESPONSES: STUDIES WITH VINYL CHLORIDE

R. P. Sharma

TABLE OF CONTENTS

I. INTRODUCTION

The problem of immunlogic testing of chemicals that are sometimes present in the industrial environment is very important. Workers are often exposed to these chemicals in concentrations far in excess to those that would be possible elsewhere in the atmosphere. Moreover, the exposure in the workplace is repetitive or chronic in nature and chemicals can get into the body via both inhalation and skin routes.

The threshold limit value (TLV) or maximum allowable concentration (MAC) for industrial chemicals are often based on sensitive toxicologic parameters. The values are generally lower than those that have been shown or suggested to produce any toxic effects. However, some cases of immunologic responses, e.g., allergic reactions, are not necessarily dose-related and even a small exposure in sensitized individuals can trigger a response. Similarly, if the chemicals in the environment are immunosuppressive, long-term exposure to these compounds may result in decreased host-defense mechanisms and lead to an increased incidence of infections or decreased ability to reject foreign cells (e.g., malignant tissues).

It is estimated that 20% of the occupational contact dermatoses are produced by allergic mechanisms. Examples of sensitizing chemicals include epoxy monomers, potassium dichromate, formaldehyde, nickel, tetramethylthiuram disulfide, mercaptobenzothiazol, etc.[1] It is often extremely difficult to distinguish between a primary irritant and a cutaneous sensitizer since marginal irritants may require a prolonged or repeated contact with the skin.

Very little emphasis has been placed on immunlogic mechanisms that are influenced by industrial chemicals. Although investigations involving immunologic testing have been conducted on individuals suffering from occupational dermatoses,[2] the findings are not conclusive. Controlled experiments need to be performed to elucidate the immunologic nature of the disease.

II. VINYL CHLORIDE DISEASE AS AN IMMUNE COMPLEX DISORDER

Ward et al.[3] were first to suggest that exposure of workers to high concentrations of vinyl chloride may result in the production of immune complexes in these individuals, and this may be a possible mechanism by which vinyl chloride may produce its toxic effects. The actions of vinyl chloride have been characterized as dermal induration, acro-osteolysis, splenomegaly, and thrombocytopenia.[4,5] Workers exposed to vinyl chloride for a long duration may also develop hepatic fibrosis associated with or leading to portal hypertension and angiosarcoma of liver.[6] Various types of tumors have been reported in animals exposed to vinyl chloride.[7]

The immunologic investigations by the above researchers[3] were conducted in fifty-eight patients that were later divided into four clinical groups. The division among these groups was based upon the severity of clinical manifestations ranging from individuals suffering with well-defined evidence of vinyl chloride disease to the patients that did not show any symptoms but were exposed to the chemical. Immunoglobulins, complement, cryo-protein, rheumatoid factor, and antitissue antibodies were determined in the serum or plasma of the exposed individuals. The peripheral lymphocytes were tested for transformation in response to phytohemagglutinin or purified protein derivative of tuberculin. In addition, T and B lymphocyte subpopulations were determined by E rosette forming cells and membrane–fluorescent cells, respectively. Biopsy specimens were evaluated by direct immunofluorescence for the presence of immunoglobulin complement, or fibrin-like substances.

The authors reported that abnormalities such as an increase of IgG, presence of mixed cryoglobulins, and in vivo conversion of both C4 and C3 were observed. The abnormalities were generally present in all cases of group 1 (severe symptoms) and the incidence of abnormalities decreased progressively in other groups. Circulating immune complexes were suggested, their frequency showing a close relationship with different clinical groups. The incidence of these immune complexes was 88% in group 1 (severe symptoms) to 0% in group 4 (asymptomatic). A high incidence of antinuclear antibodies was also shown in group 1. A decrease in T cell population with a slight increase in B cells was reported in all groups. A variable degree of reduction in the responses of lymphocytes to tuberculin protein or phytohemagglutinin was observed in cultures. Biopsy studies showed aggregates of immune complexes adherent to the vascular endothelium in the lumen of vessels in skin, muscle, and lung.

The presence of hyperimmunoglobinemia, cryoglobulinemia, and cryofibrinogenemia along with antitissue antibodies were strongly suggestive of immune-complex disorders in vinyl chloride syndrome. The immunofluorescence studies of biopsy material further confirmed the presence of circulating immune complexes. The authors suggested that a reactive metabolite of vinyl chloride may bind with a tissue protein, rendering it antigenic. The macromolecular binding of vinyl chloride in hepatic tissue has been demonstrated.[8,9]

Page et al.[10] reported elevated levels of carcino-embryonic antigen (CEA) levels in workers exposed to vinyl chloride. This increase was reported in individuals not showing any definite liver disease and suggested that this measurement may be used as a diagnostic aid.

III. LYMPHOCYTE STIMULATION BY VINYL CHLORIDE

Thurman et al.[11] have recently reported on the effect of vinyl chloride in lymphocytes obtained from mice exposed to 500 ppm of this chemical for various periods. The chemical was fatal to these mice at a concentration of 1000 ppm during a 7 hr exposure resulting in 90% mortality within 18 hr. Vinyl chloride at 1000 ppm concentration had no effect on the immune reactivity of lymphocytes obtained from various lymphatic organs when these cells were cultured in a vinyl chloride atmosphere. Exposure of mice to 500 ppm vinyl chloride for 7 hr produced inconsistent results when their lymphocytes were cultured in vitro in the presence of various mitogenic agents. Splenic lymphocytes from the exposed animals showed a decreased response to mitogenic agents when the cells were obtained one day after the exposure. Three days after vinyl chloride exposure, 72 hr-cultures in the presence of Phytohemagglutinin-P (PHAP) showed a large stimulation, whereas no effect was observed after 14 days of exposure. In mixed splenic lymphocyte cultures, a consistent stimulation was found in exposed animals as compared to untreated controls at 14 days after vinyl chloride exposure. Similar inconsistencies or noneffects were seen in lymphocytes from lymph nodes or thymus at various periods after a single day exposure to vinyl chloride. The authors suggested that acute exposure to vinyl chloride caused no deleterious effects on the immunological system of mice. A summary of the effects of vinyl chloride exposure along with other industrial chemicals are listed in Table 1.

Sharma and Gehring[12] exposed mice to different levels of vinyl chloride, in the range of 10—1000 ppm, 6 hr/day, 5 days/week up to 8 weeks. Such exposure to vinyl chloride did not produce any effect on body weight, organ weight, and organ/body weight ratios, except an enlargement of spleen was observed at 2 and 4 weeks after the exposure of mice to 1000 ppm vinyl chloride. When the splenic lymphocytes from these animals were cultured after 2, 4 or 8 weeks of exposure, a dose- and time-dependent stimulation of lymphocyte transformation was observed. At the end of 2 weeks of exposure, the stim-

Table 1
SUMMARY OF THE EFFECTS OF VARIOUS COMPOUNDS ON THE IMMUNOLOGICAL RESPONSITIVITY OF LYMPHOCYTES

Compound	Murine In vitro	Murine In vivo	Human In vitro
Control compounds			
Azathioprine	ND[a]	ND	Nonspecifically cytotoxic at 100 μg/mℓ
Hydrocortisone acetate	More lymphotoxic to PHA-responsive cells than Con A-responsive cells; nonspecifically cytotoxic at 50 μg/mℓ or greater	ND	ND
TEM	Nonspecifically cytotoxic at concentrations as low as 50 μg/mℓ	ND	Nonspecifically cytotoxic at concentrations as low as 0.1 μg/mℓ
Chemicals			
Benzene	ND	ND	Nonspecifically cytotoxic at 2.5%; little or no effect at 1% and lower
Dioxane	Enhancement of B cell responses while inhibitory to T cell responses; lymphotoxic at concentrations greater than 1%	Very little immunosuppression potency below lethal dosage levels	Some enhancement of PHA-P responses at 2.5% with little effect at lower concentrations
TDI	ND	May be stimulatory through antigenic properties; inhibitory to responses to T cell mitogens in spleen and lymph node	Low concentrations stimulated some lymphocyte proliferation as in a reaction to antigen; otherwise mildly and nonspecifically immunosuppressive
Vinylidene chloride	ND	ND	No consistent effect at concentrations up to 2.5%
Vinyl chloride	ND	No demonstrable immunosuppressive effect even at toxic doses (500 ppm, 7 hr)	ND
Ethylenimine	Nonspecifically cytotoxic at levels as low as 20 μg/well; augmented PHA-P responses at 4 and 0.4 μg/well	ND	Nonspecifically cytotoxic at concentrations as low as 3 μg/well

Epichlorohydrin	Somewhat more cytotoxic to B cells at doses less than 150 μg/well, whereas it is nonspecifically cytotoxic at 300 μg/well	ND	Nonspecifically cytotoxic at 60 μg/well; at lower concentrations it is suppressive to the Con A and PWM response and not to the PHA-P response

[a] ND, not done.

(From Thurman, G. B., Simms, B. G., Goldstein, A. L., and Kilian, D. J., *Toxicol. Appl. Pharmacol.*, 44, 617, 1978. With permission.)

ulation was seen only at the highest concentration of exposure, i.e., 1000 ppm vinyl chloride. Four weeks after the exposure was started, there was stimulation of lymphocyte transformation seen in all groups, the effect increasing at 10 and 100 ppm of vinyl chloride, but showing a slight decline at 1000 ppm vinyl chloride. The mice exposed to 1000 ppm vinyl chloride, however, showed a significant increase over the respective controls. After 8 weeks of exposure, the effect was similar to that observed at the 4-week period. However, the decline at the highest level was more pronounced at the 8-week period. Again, the lymphocyte transformation at the highest level of vinyl chloride exposure was higher than that observed in respective controls (Figure 1). The stimulation of splenic lymphocyte transformation was seen in cultures without any mitogen and also in the presence of optimal amounts of phytohemagglutinin or pokeweed mitogen. The stimulation indexes of splenic lymphocytes by the two phytomitogens were increased severalfold in vinyl chloride-exposed mice. It appeared that the exposure to vinyl chloride stimulated splenic lymphocyte transformation both in unstimulated cultures and in the presence of mitogenic stimulants. However, the effects were not dose-related when the concentration of vinyl chloride was high.

A similar effect was also seen in rabbits[13] when they were exposed to 10, 100 and 1000 ppm of vinyl chloride for 8 weeks. These animals showed an enlargement of thymus at the highest exposure level indicating stimulation of immune responses. No enlargement of the spleen was observed. The animals were inoculated with a mixture of an antigen (tetanus toxoid and Freunds complete adjuvant) at 4 and 6 weeks during the exposure, but no consistent effect on serum antitetanus titers, skin reactivity to tuberculin or the number of antibody producing cells (Plasma cells) in popliteal lymph node was seen in relation to vinyl chloride exposure. When the splenic lymphocytes from these animals were cultured, their DNA synthesis without any mitogen was significantly increased in cells obtained from animals exposed to 10 and 100 ppm of vinyl chloride. The increase at the 1000 ppm level was not significant. In these animals the effects of mitogenic stimulation (phytohemagglutinin and pokeweed mitogen) were not consistent, perhaps because the lymphocytes were already stimulated in vivo by antigenic challenge. The findings in rabbit studies supported the observations that low levels of vinyl chloride exposure in mice caused an enhancement of immune responsivity of splenic lymphocytes. The effects of chronic exposure to vinyl chloride were similar to those observed when the murine splenic lymphocytes were cultured for 72 hr in the presence of phytohemagglutinin 3 weeks after a single acute exposure.[11]

The enhancement of immunological reactivity in vinyl chloride-exposed animals is consistent with the presence of circulating immune complexes in patients with vinyl chloride disease syndrome as reported by Ward et al.[3] Whether such immune complexes are produced as a result of autoimmune phenomena in response to an altered body protein or to a haptenic conjugate of vinyl chloride is not known. It is also possible that the stimulation of immune reactivity in exposed workers results in the formation of immune complexes against some usual antigens that may not show any effect in normal individuals.

IV. VINYL CHLORIDE METABOLISM AND LYMPHOCYTE TRANSFORMATION

Based on the findings stated above, Sharma and Gehring[12] investigated the role of vinyl chloride metabolism on stimulated lymphocyte transformation in mice. Since the observed alterations in lymphocyte mitosis were not time- and dose-related, it was hypothesized that a reactive metabolite of vinyl chloride, rather than the parent compound itself, may be responsible for producing immunologic effects. Vinyl chloride is metabo-

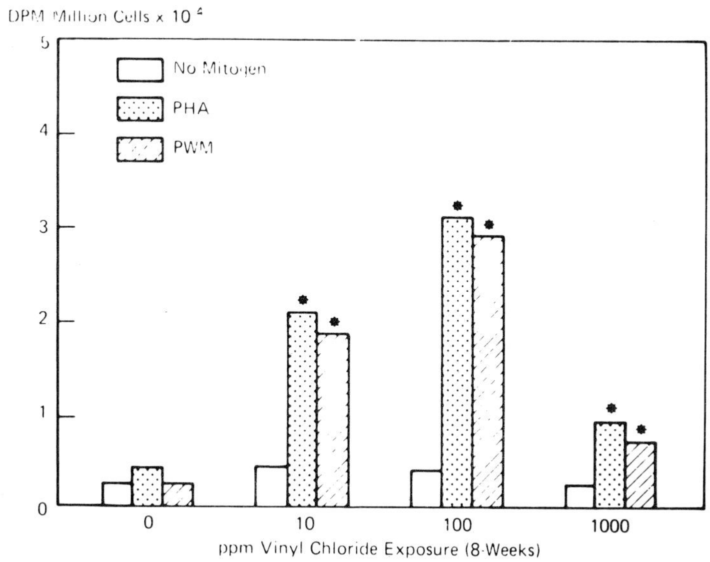

FIGURE 1. Stimulation of splenic lymphocyte transformation in 72 hr cultures with or without the presence of phytohemagglutinin and pokeweek mitogen. The values are average of four animals in each case. Astericks (*) indicate a significant difference from the respective coantrol value at $p < 0.05$. Reproduced with permissi

lized through the epoxide intermediate chloroethylene epoxide,[14,15] which is believed to be a potent alkylating agent. Since lymphocyte transformation represents increased mitotic activity of these cells and involves increased synthesis of deoxyribonucleic acid (DNA), this effect may be mediated through the reaction of this epoxide metabolite with critical DNA receptors. The authors thus studied the effect of altered vinyl chloride metabolism on the splenic lymphocyte transformation.

Mice were treated with ethanol and phenobarbital just prior to their daily exposures with 1000 ppm vinyl chloride, 6 hr/day for 5 days, and their spleens harvested 2 days after the last exposure. Appropriate saline-treated controls and animals treated with ethanol and phenobarbital were exposed simultaneously to room air in identical chambers. Ethanol is a known inhibitor of vinyl chloride metabolism. Treatment with ethanol decreased the vinyl chloride-induced stimulation of splenic lymphocyte transformation. The effect of ethanol on the immune reactivity of these lymphocytes was taken into consideration; comparisons were made between ethanol-treated groups exposed to either vinyl chloride or room air. The stimulation of lymphocyte transformation by exposure to vinyl chloride was seen in saline-treated groups. The results suggested that decreasing the metabolizing capacity of the animal for vinyl chloride reduced the immunostimulatory effects and hence these effects were mediated via one of its active metabolites.

Treatment of mice with phenobarbital also produced similar results. It has been reported that vinyl chloride metabolism is not induced in phenobarbital-treated microsomal systems.[8] Although the rate of vinyl chloride metabolism is not increased, the treatment with phenobarbital increased its covalent binding in the hepatic tissue.[9] Treatment of mice with phenobarbital prior to vinyl chloride exposure reduced the lymphocyte transformation in spleen. The findings support the view that there was an increased macromolecular binding of the vinyl chloride metabolite in tissues thus reducing its effective concentration on cells of the immune system.

The incubation of splenic lymphocyte cultures in a vinyl chloride atmosphere did not produce any effect on the transformation of cells. The results involving the liver metabolizing systems in the culture medium were not conclusive since the presence of liver proteins caused a marked inhibition of lymphocyte transformation. Similarly, the two known metabolites of vinyl chloride, thiodiglycolic acid and *N*-acetyl-*S*-(hydroxyethyl) cystein,[16] when added directly to the culture medium did not provide conclusive results. Oral administration of thiodiglycolic acid in mice, however, produced a dose-related stimulation of splenic lymphocyte transformation[16] similar to the one observed with vinyl chloride exposure.

V. LYMPHOCYTE RESPONSES IN VINYL CHLORIDE-EXPOSED WORKERS

Fortwengler et al.[17] have reported the transformation of circulating lympocytes in vinyl chloride-exposed workers. Some of these workers had a diagnosed liver disease. The stimulation of peripheral lymphocytes by phytohemagglutinin in cultures was not different in vinyl chloride-exposed individuals when compared to a control group. The stimulation of lymphocyte transformation by the tumor-associated antigen and by normal tissue antigen was somewhat depressed when lymphocytes were collected from the vinyl chloride-exposed workers. The authors suggested that there was a lower overall lymphocytes responsiveness in chemical workers. The observation was in contrast to that noticed in animals after a repeated but short-term exposure to vinyl chloride. However, it may be consistent with the animal data where the lymphocytes showed declining stimulation indices when obtained from the animals exposed to 1000 ppm vinyl chloride for 8 weeks.[12] It may also be noted that the vinyl chloride-exposed workers may or may not have liver–associated diseases whereas no liver–associated condition was observed in animals after an 8-week exposure.

VI. OTHER RELATED INDUSTRIAL CHEMICALS

A study of the effects of a number of industrial chemicals associated with the plastic industry has been conducted by Thurman et al.[11] These workers investigated the effect of various chemicals on lymphocyte transformation of cells obtained from various lymphoid organs (spleen, thymus, lymph node) in mice exposed to these chemicals. The effects of in vitro addition of these chemicals to cultures of the cells mentioned above and to cultures of human peripheral lymphocytes were studied. The results are summarized in Table 1.

The data shown in Table 1 indicate that various chemicals may have both immunostimulatory and inhibitory properties. The effects are often dose-related. For example, dioxane when added directly to the cultures, showed a slight stimulation of lymphocyte transformation at very low concentrations, while it was lymphotoxic at high concentrations. This chemical did not show a consistent effect after an in vivo administration. The data presented by the above authors, however, indicated that animals injected with 0.5 mℓ of 0.1 or 1% dioxane in saline for 7 days sometimes showed a stimulation of lymphocyte transformation, whereas higher dose levels were often inhibitory. Similarly, ethylenimine showed an augmented response at 0.4 and 4 μg/culture when added to mice lymphocytes while higher concentration of this chemical showed a cytotoxic effect. Preliminary studies have been conducted on animals exposed to various chemicals and after in vitro addition of the chemicals in cultures. The results of these studies are presented in Volume II, Chapter 7.

VII. FUTURE NEEDS

It appears that very little attention has been devoted to the immunologic testing of chemicals that are often present in the industrial environment. Although a limited number of the total population is exposed to these chemicals, the exposures are usually prolonged, ranging up to several years, and the concentrations in the environment may be relatively high when compared to the chemicals present in the outside environment.

Results of a number of studies have suggested that some industrial chemicals have a positive or negative influence on the immune reactivity of the exposed individuals. The effects may lead to allergic sensitization of individuals and the possibility of autoimmune diseases caused by chronic damage to organs and tissues. In the case of immunosuppression this may lead to increased sensitivity to infections and interference with prophylactic immunization. In an industrial environment the alteration of immune function may be important since various physical irritants are usually present. For example, the sensitivity of individuals to respiratory infections will be further increased if there is an effective immunosuppression by chemical exposure and a simultaneous inhalation of obviously innocuous chemical substances that may cause physical lung damage is present. The same may also be true if there was a simultaneous exposure to very small amounts of a weak chemical carcinogen. The incidence of a carcinogenic effect may be sufficiently altered by the manipulation of immune functions.

There is an increased need to further investigate the mechanisms involved in the modification of immune responses, once the chemicals are shown to have an effect on such systems. Studies leading to the cellular and molecular mechanisms can be helpful in predicting the effects of new chemicals and in advocating the preventive measures in case of excessive exposures to harmful chemicals.

Apart from the experimental studies involving industrial chemicals, the exposure to workers provides an ideal situation for studying their effects on the human immune responses. In most cases the workers are routinely checked for their health status and inclusion of some of the immunological parameters will be of value, particularly for the chemicals that are suspected of producing alterations of this system. For example, differential quantitative estimation of immunoglobulins and evaluation of lymphocyte function can be performed. These studies together with the epidemiological data obtained on the incidence of carcinogenesis may at some stage provide information associating the immune-surveillance mechanisms with actual cancer production.

REFERENCES

1. **Birmingham, D. J.,** Dermatoses, in, Occupational Diseases: Guide to Their Recognition, Publ. No. 77-181, U.S. Department of Health, Education and Welfare, U.S. Government Printing Office, Washington, D.C., 1977, 78.
2. **Avery, S. B., Stetsen, D. M., Pan, P. M., and Mathews, K. P.,** Immunological investigation of individuals with toluene diisocyanate asthma, *Clin. Exp. Immunol.,* 4, 585, 1969.
3. **Ward, A. M., Udnoon, S., Watkins, J., Walker, A. E., and Darke, C. S.,** Immunological mechanisms in the pathogenesis of vinyl chloride disease, *Br. Med. J.,* 1, 936, 1976.
4. **Harris, D. K. and Adams, W. G. F.,** Acroosteolysis occurring in men engaged in the polymerization of vinyl chloride, *Br. Med. J.,* 3, 712, 1967.
5. **Lange, C. E., Juhe, S., Stein, G., and Veltman, G.,** The so-called vinyl chloride disease, an occupational systemic sclerosis? *Int. Arch. Arbeitzmed.,* 32, 1, 1974.

6. **Berk, P. D., Martin, J. F., Young, R. S., Creech, J., Salikoff, I. J., Falk, H., Watanabe, P., Popper, H., and Thomas, L.,** Vinyl chloride associated liver disease. *Ann. Intern. Med.*, 84, 717, 1976.
7. **Maltoni, S. and LeFemine, G.,** Carcinogenecity bioassays of vinyl chloride. I. Research plan and early results, *Environ. Res.*, 7, 387, 1974.
8. **Kappas, H., Bolt, H. M., Buchler, A., and Bolt, W.,** Liver microsomal uptake of ^{14}C vinyl chloride and transformation to protein alkylating metabolites in vitro, *Toxicol. Appl. Pharmacol.*, 37, 461, 1976.
9. **Watanabe, P. G., Zempel, J. A., Pegg, D. G. and Gehring, P. J.,** Hepatic macromolecular bindng following exposure to vinyl chloride, *Toxicol, Appl. Pharmacol.*, 44, 571, 1978.
10. **Page, M., Teriault, L. and Delorme, F.,** Elevated CEA levels in polyvinyl chloride workers, *Biomedicine*, 25, 279, 1976.
11. **Thurman, G. B., Simms, B. G., Goldstein, A. L. and Kilian, D. J.,** The effects of organic compounds used in the manufacture of plastics on the responsivity of murine and human lymphocytes, *Toxicol. Appl. Pharmacol.*, 44, 617, 1978.
12. **Sharma, R. P. and Gehring, P. J.,** Immunologic effects of vinyl chloride in mice, *Ann. N.Y. Acad. Sci.*, In Press.
13. **Sharma, R. P., Yakel, H. O. and Gehring, P. J.,** Immunotoxicologic studies with vinyl chloride in rabbits and mice, *Int. J. Immunopharmacol.*, In Press, 1981.
14. **Hefner, R. E., Watanabe, P. G. and Gehring, P. J.,** Preliminary studies of the fate of inhaled vinyl chloride monomers (VCM) in rats, *Ann. N.Y. Acad. Sci.*, 246, 135, 1975.
15. **Barbin, A., Bresil, H., Croisg, P., Jacquoignon, P., Malaveille, G., Montesano, R. and Bartsch, H.,** Liver microsome mediated formation of alkylating agents from vinyl bromide and vinyl chloride, *Biochem. Biophys. Res. Commun.*, 67, 596, 1975.
16. **Sharma, R. P. and Gehring, P. J.,** Unpublished data.
17. **Fortwengler, H. P., Deva, M. E., Tamburro, C. H. and Espinosa, E.,** Lymphocyte transformation tests in vinyl chloride (VC) workers, *Fed. Proc. Fed. Am. Soc. Exp. Biol.*, 37, 362, 1978.

Chapter 9

EFFECTS OF TETRACHLORODIBENZO-*p*-DIOXIN (TCDD) ON IMMUNOLOGIC SYSTEMS

R. P. Sharma

TABLE OF CONTENTS

I. INTRODUCTION

Tetrachlorodibenzo-*p*-dioxin (TCDD) is one of the most toxic manmade chemicals.[1] It is present as a contaminant formed during the production of trichlorophenols prior to subsequent manufacture of the herbicide, 2,4,5-trichlorophenoxyacetic acid (2,4,5-T). It has also been found in other chlorophenols and related compounds.[2,3] The synthesis of TCDD during chemical manufacturing processes is illustrated in Figure 1.

TCDD produces toxic effects in various mammalian species, the toxic manifestations often depend on the species. Guinea pigs are very sensitive to the toxic effects of TCDD, the single dose LD_{50} for this chemical being <1 μg/kg body weight. The LD_{50} value for mice and rabbits is ~ 100 μg/kg. The toxic effects of the chemical include hepatic damage,[4] thymic atrophy,[5,6] hematological alterations[7] and teratologic effects[8] in various species. It has been suggested that TCDD may be the causative factor for chloracne produced in exposed workers in 2,4,5-T herbicide manufacturing.

A consistent toxic effect of TCDD in various test animals is damage to the thymus gland. A dose-related depletion of thymocytes from this organ leading to cortical atrophy and thymic involution has been described in various species of laboratory animals. Subsequent to this finding, a number of studies involving possible immunosuppressive effects of this chemical have been performed and will be summarized in this report.

II. EFFECT OF TCDD ON THYMUS AND OTHER ORGANS

Buu-Hoi et al.[5] were the first to suggest that sublethal doses of TCDD produced thymus atrophy and proposed that this organ along with liver and heart were the target organs of dioxin toxicity. Single or repeated toxic doses of TCDD caused a decrease in body weight and several vital organs and often a reduction in the organ/body weight ratios. One exception to this was the weight of liver, which is generally increased by TCDD treatment. TCDD is a potent inducer of liver microsomal and related enzymes.[9] It also produces liver hypertrophy, generally associated with degenerative and necrotic lesions in this organ.

The effects of TCDD exposure on various species of laboratory animals together with its effect on body weight are summarized in Table 1. As indicated in Table 1, TCDD caused a reduction of body weight in guinea pigs, rats, mice, rabbits and monkeys. Guinea pigs showed the greatest sensitivity to TCDD, their weight reduction being obvious at 0.2 μg/kg/week for 8 weeks. Rats and mice, on the other hand, are relatively resistant to the effects of TCDD; the effect on body or organ weight appeared when a single or cumulative dose of this chemical was 100 μg/kg or more. In all species, a consistent reduction in thymus weight was seen. This is often associated with atrophy of the thymic cortex subsequent to the gradual depletion of lymphocytes in this area at low doses of TCDD. Depletion of thymocytes in the thymic cortex of mice is shown in Figure 2.

III. IMMUNOSUPPRESSIVE EFFECTS OF TCDD IN LABORATORY ANIMALS

Table 2 summarizes the representative studies performed on the immunosuppressive effects of TCDD. Vos and co-workers[6] reported the effects of TCDD on the immune system of guinea pigs, rats, and mice. Several tests were employed in these three species and the authors concluded that the effect of TCDD was primarily on the cell-mediated immune mechanisms of these animals.

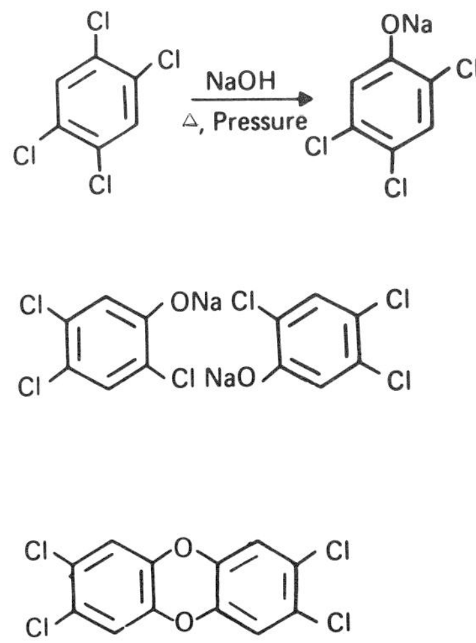

TCDD

FIGURE 1. Possible mechanism of synthesis of TCDD in the manufacture of chlorophenols.

Table 1
SENSITIVITY OF VARIOUS SPECIES OF LABORATORY ANIMALS TO TETRACHLORODIBENZO-*p*-DIOXIN (TCDD): EFFECTS ON BODY WEIGHT AND ORGANS RELATED TO IMMUNE SYSTEM[a]

Species	Dose range used	Organ or body weight	Effect observed	Ref.
Guinea pig	0.008—2 μg/kg once a week for 8 weeks	Body weight	Decreased at ≥0.2 μg/kg	6
		Thymus weight	Decreased at ≥0.04 μg/kg	
		Spleen weight	Not affected	
Rat	0.2—5 μg/kg once a week for 6 weeks	Body weight	Decreased at the highest dose	6
		Thymus weight and thymus/body weight	Decreased at the highest dose	
		Spleen/body weight	Increased at the highest dose	
Mice	0.2—25 μg/kg once a week for 4 weeks	Growth rate	Decreased at the highest dose	6
		Thymus weight and its ratio to body weight	Decreased at ≥5 μg/kg dose	
Mice	0.2—25 μg/kg once a week for 2 or 6 weeks	Weight gain	Decreased at 5 and 25 μg/kg dose at 2 weeks, but at 25 μg/kg at 6 weeks	10
		Thymus weight and its ratio to body weight	Decreased at ≥1 μg/kg dose at both periods	
Rat	0.001—1 μg/kg/day daily for 13 weeks	Body and organ weights	Reduced at ≥0.1 μg/kg, except liver showed increase	11

Table 1 (continued)
SENSITIVITY OF VARIOUS SPECIES OF LABORATORY ANIMALS TO TETRACHLORODIBENZO-*p*-DIOXIN (TCDD): EFFECTS ON BODY WEIGHT AND ORGANS RELATED TO IMMUNE SYSTEM[a]

Species	Dose range used	Organ or body weight	Effect observed	Ref.
Mice	1.5 and 50 μg/kg weekly for 4 weeks	Body, thymus and spleen weight	All reduced at 50 μg/kg dose	12
Mice	0.01—10 μg/kg weekly for 2-8 weeks	Thymus weight	Decreased at 1 μg/kg after 2 weeks	13
		Spleen	Increase at 0.1 and 1 μg/kg after 2 weeks	
Rabbits	0.01—10 μg/kg weekly for 10 weeks	Thymus and its ratio to body weight	Decreased at the highest dose	14
		Adrenals weight	Decreased at the highest dose	
		Popliteal lymph node	Decreased at the highest dose	
Monkey	70 and 350 μg/kg single oral dose	Body weight	Decreased	15
		Relative organ weights	Increased except Thymus reduced	

[a] In many reports a dose-related increase in liver weight was reported. Some of the experiments reported also involved a challenge with an antigen to evaluate immune responsiveness.

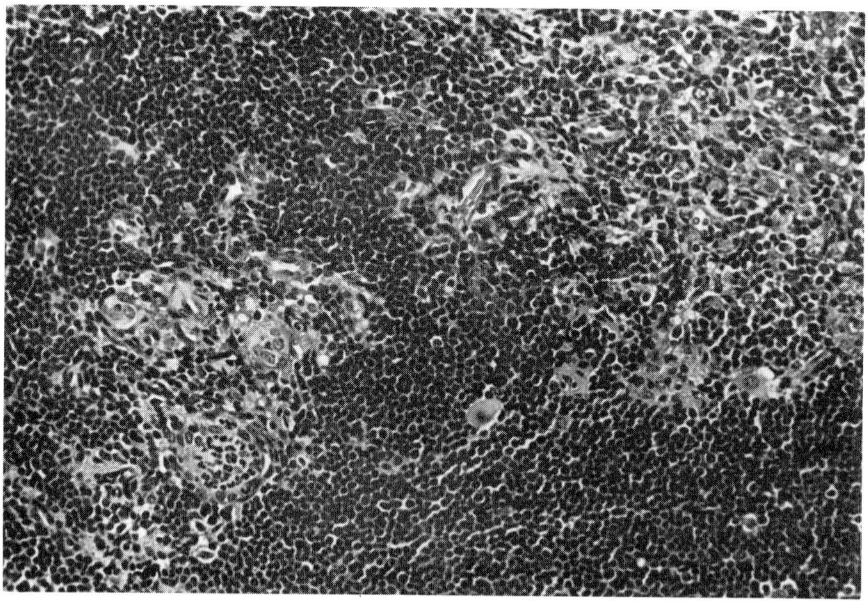

FIGURE 2. Depletion of thymocytes from the cortical area of a mouse thymus after treatment with TCDD.

Table 2
SELECTED IMMUNOSUPPRESSIVE EFFECTS OF TETRACHLORODIBENZO-*p*-DIOXIN (TCDD)

Species	Dose	Effects observed	Ref.
Guinea pigs	0.008—0.2 μg/kg weekly × 8	Primary antitoxin to tetanus toxoid increased at 0.008 and 0.04 μg/kg levels but secondary response decreased at 0.2 μg/kg dose Delayed hypersensitivity to tuberculin decreased at 0.04 and 2 μg/kg Blood leukocytes decreased at 0.04 μg/kg and lymphocytes at all treatment levels	6
Rats	0.2—5 μg/kg weekly × 6	No effect on peripheral total leukocytes or lymphocytes Skin reactivity to tuberculin not affected	6
Mice	0.2—5 μg/kg weekly × 4	Graft vs. host activity of spleen cells reduced at 5 μg/kg dose	6
Mice	0.5—20 μg/kg weekly × 4	Significant increase in mortality to Salmonella infection but no effect on pseudorabies virus infectivity	17
Mice	0.2—25 μg/kg	Increased neutrophils at the highest dose after 2 weeks; decreased hemoglobin and corpuscular volume at 25 μg/kg dose after 6 weeks; a decrease in globulin concentrations at various dose levels	10
Mice	1.5—50 μg/kg weekly × 4	Increased sensitivity to *Escherichia coli* endotoxin at ≥5 μg/kg dose, no effect on nonspecific phagocytosis	12
Mice	0.01—10 μg/kg weekly × 8, challenged with tetanus toxoid	Antitetanus titers decreased at 10 μg/kg dose	14
Rabbits	0.01—10 μg/kg weekly × 8, challenged with antigens	Antitetanus titers decreased at ≥0.1 μg/kg dose; plasma cells in lymph nodes decreased at ≥1 μg/kg/week and skin reactivity decreased at all dose levels	14

Guinea pigs treated with 1 μg/kg of TCDD per week either died or were moribund after 4 doses. At this dose and also at small doses (0.008, 0.04, and 0.2 μg/kg), guinea pigs showed severe loss of body weight, depletion of the lymphoid organs, particularly thymus, and lymphopenia. At sublethal doses the effects were primarily on the thymus. The weights of other lymphoid organs, such as spleen, cervical lymph nodes, and popliteal lymph nodes, were not affected. Adrenals showed a slight enlargement at the 0.2 μg/kg dose level. Serum cortiol and corticosterone values were not influenced by the TCDD treatment. No microscopic lesions were apparent in any of the lymphoid organs upon dosing with up to 0.2 μg TCDD per kg per week, however, atrophy of the thymic cortex occurred.

In selected experiments, the treated and control animals were injected with a subcutaneous dose of tetanus toxoid or an oil suspension of killed *Mycobacterium tuberculosis*. Seven days after the tetanus toxoid injection, there was a small but significant increase in the serum antitoxin levels at 0.008 and 0.04 μg/kg dose levels. The animals were challenged again by a second dose of tetanus toxoid 2 weeks after the first challenge to evaluate the secondary response. One and two weeks after the second dose, the guinea pigs treated with 0.2 μg TCDD per kg per week had significantly lower tetanus antitoxin titers. The animals challenged with *M. tuberculosis* were tested for their skin reactivity 12 and 19 days later by intradermal tuberculin injections. Both skin diameter and skin thickness of the reaction site were significantly decreased, the former being significant at the 0.04 μg/kg dose level.

Female albino rats were treated orally with 0.2, 1, and 5 μg/kg of TCDD once a week for 6 weeks. All animals survived the experimental period. The body weight and thymus weights were reduced at the highest dose level and adrenal weights were reduced at the 1 and 5 μg/kg level. The relative thymus weight (organ/body weight ratio) was approximately half that of the control animals at the 5 μg/kg dose level, whereas at the same dose level, the relative spleen weights were significantly increased. The total peripheral leukocyte and lymphocyte numbers did not show a significant TCDD-related effect as observed in guinea pigs. Skin reactivity of killed *M. tuberculosis*-challenged rats to a tuberculin was not affected at any TCDD level.

Graft vs. host (GVH) activity of mice was evaluated after 0.2, 1, 5, and 25 μg/TCDD per kg per week for 4 weeks. The absolute and relative thymus weights were decreased in groups treated with $\geq$5 μg TCDD/kg. The GVH reaction (described later in Volume II, Chapter 5) is characterized by the tolerance of immunocompetent cells by a hybrid recipient. Single-cell suspensions of spleens from the treated mice were inoculated into the foot-pads of hybrid recipient mice. The enlarged lymph node of the injected leg (right popliteal node) was compared to the uninjected leg and graft vs. host activity ratios computed. The average ratio in control animals was found to be approximately 6, and a gradual TCDD-related reduction in GVH activity was observed. The reported GVH ratio for cells from mice injected with 5 μg/kg/week of TCDD was about 2, a significant reduction from the control value.

On the basis of the results summarized above, the authors concluded that TCDD suppressed the cell-mediated immunity in guinea pigs and mice. The humoral immunity in guinea pigs was also slightly suppressed. The effects were not so marked in rats. In the sensitive species, the immunologic effects were probably not caused through other endocrine mechanisms.

IV. SUPPRESSION OF CELLULAR IMMUNITY BY MATERNAL TREATMENT

Vos and Moore[16] have reported the effects of maternal TCDD exposure on the offspring of rats and mice. Complicated experimental designs employing prenatal exposure, postnatal exposure of mothers, or a continued prenatal through postnatal exposure were carried out. The immunological reactivity of newborn animals or of suckling rats and mice were evaluated by various test procedures. The representative results of these studies are summarized in Table 3.

Female pregnant rats were treated orally with 1 or 5 μg TCDD per kg body weight on day 11 and 18 of gestation. The weights of 1-day-old pups from mothers treated with 5 μg/kg level were significantly reduced. At this dose level, reduced weights of thymus and spleen were also observed. Most of the pups in the high treatment group died within 25 days after birth. The newborn animals from mothers given 1 μg/kg dose level were

Table 3
IMMUNOSUPPRESSIVE EFFECT OF TETRACHLORODIBENZO-*p*-DIOXIN IN NEWBORN RATS AND MICE BY MATERNAL PRENATAL AND/OR POSTNATAL TREATMENT

Species	Dose and schedule	Parameters observed and effects reported
Rat	1 or 5 μg/kg on day 11 and 18 of gestation	A reduction in body, thymus and spleen weights of 1-day-old pups at 5 μg/kg dose
	1 μg/kg prenatally on 11 and 18 days of gestation, and 4, 11, and 18 days postnatal	Body, thymus and adrenal weights decreased in 25-day-old rats
	5 μg/kg postnatally on 4, 11, and 18 days	Body, thymus and spleen weights decreased in 25-day-old rats
	Pre- and postnatally as described above	The responsiveness of spleen cells to PHA not influenced but the responsiveness expressed as whole spleen decreased; no effect on GVH response
	Postnatally only as described above	PHA responsiveness of spleen cells decreased at 5 μg/kg dose; GVH response decreased; PHA and Con A response in thymus cells decreased
	5 μg/kg postnatally on 4, 11, and 18 days	Rejection time for tail-skin grafts increased
Mice	2 and 5 μg/kg on 14 and 17 days of gestation and postnatally on day 1, 8, and 15	Rejection time for heterologous tail-skin graft increased at both dose levels
Mice	1-month-old mice treated with 1, 5, and 25 μg/kg weekly doses for 4 weeks	Body weight decreased at the highest dose, thymus weight decreased at 5 and 25 μg/kg dose levels; PHA responsiveness of splenic cells decreased and slight decrease in GVH activity noticed
	4-month-old mice treated with 1, 5, and 25 μg/kg weekly for 6 weeks	A decrease in body weight at the highest dose, and that of thymus at all treated levels; no effect on splenic responsiveness to PHA or GHV activity

Based on the results reported by Vos and Moore, *Int. Arch. Allergy,* 47, 777, 1974.

further treated with the same dose of TCDD administered to mothers on day 4, 11 and 18. Additional groups of suckling rats were exposed to TCDD postnatally by oral treatment of mothers with 5 μg/kg dose. Reduction in body, thymus, spleen, and adrenal weights were observed in different groups at 25 days of age. Splenic lymphocytes of rats exposed postnatally to 5 μg/kg level showed a decrease in phytohemagglutinin (PHA)-induced DNA synthesis. This effect was not observed in animals exposed pre- and postnatally to 1 μg TCDD per kg. Since the spleen weights were considerably reduced, the PHA-responsiveness was decreased in both experiments when expressed on the total spleen basis.

Similar effects were observed on graft-vs.-host activity of spleen cells from 25-day–old pre- and/or postnatally exposed rats. The weights of popliteal lymph nodes in incompatible recipient rats were not reduced when compared to controls in animals treated pre- and postnatally with 1 μg TCDD per kg. The animals treated with 5 μg/kg postnatally, however, showed a significant decrease in GVH activity of spleen cells.

The thymocytes from postnatally exposed male rats to 5 μg/kg level of TCDD showed a significant reduction of thymidine incorporation in cultures in the presence of PHA. The DNA synthesis in response to concanavalin A (Con A) was, however, not reduced in thymocytes, although a decrease was seen if the data were expressed on the basis of total thymus.

When the rats were grafted with skin from heterologous donors (on the tail), the animals exposed postnatally showed a significant increase in the rejection time of the grafts. Similar increases were observed in pre- and postnatally-exposed mice whose mothers were treated with 2 or 5 μg TCDD per kg on days 14 and 17 of gestation and day 1, 8, and 15 after birth.

In the results summarized above, the authors reported the insensitivity of 4-month old mice to TCDD treatment. One-month old mice treated with 4 weekly doses of 25 μg TCDD per kg showed a decreased responsiveness of their splenic lymphocytes to PHA, whereas 5-month old animals failed to show this effect after 6 weekly doses.

In their conclusion, Vos and Moore[16] suggested that both mice and rats show a depressed cellular immunity but the effects are largely age-dependent. A considerable suppression of cell-mediated immune mechanisms can be produced in newborns through the treatment of their mothers during gestation and nursing periods. Exposure of animals via pre- and postnatal treatment produced a condition that was similar to neonatal thymectomy. The authors speculated that the degree of such an immune-depression may contribute to the death of exposed animals and the mechanism is not related to the hepatic damage or other stress-producing syndromes.

V. SUSCEPTIBILITY OF TCDD-TREATED ANIMALS TO BACTERIAL VS. VIRAL INFECTIONS

Thigpen et al.[17] challenged groups of mice treated orally with TCDD to either *Salmonella bern* or *Herpesvirus suis.* In two separate experiments the animals were exposed to TCDD levels ranging from 0.5 to 20 μg/kg once every week for 4 weeks. The animals were challenged with the infectious agents one day after the 4th dose of TCDD. In none of the above groups did treatment with TCDD produce any appreciable change in body weight or growth rate of animals. Treatment of mice with TCDD reduced the time of death after the bacterial challenge and also increased the mortality to *S. bern.* The decrease in time before the death occurred was significant at ≥ 5 μg/kg dose level whereas the increased mortality was obvious at the TCDD treatment level of 1 μg/kg. The challenge of similar animals to *H. suis* influenced neither the period of death after the injection with this virus, nor affected the mortality rate. The authors concluded that the treatment with TCDD had a differential effect on bacterial vs. viral challenge and this difference may be accounted for by some unspecified host-defense factors. The possibility of alterations in phagocytic cell-function or in the interaction of T cells with phagocytic cells was suggested.

VI. ENDOTOXIN HYPERSENSITIVITY AND TREATMENT OF MICE WITH TCDD

Vos and co-workers[12] have reported on the response of young mice to *Escherichia coli* endotoxin after TCDD treatment. In two separate experiments, 3 to 4 week old mice were orally administered, once a week for 4 weeks, 0, 1.5, 5, 15, or 50 μg TCDD per kg. Forty-eight hours after the final dose, the animals were injected intravenously with 10, 20, 100, 250, or 500 μg of endotoxin and their mortality observed. In another experiment, the mortality to the endotoxin was studied after a single oral dose of 100 μg TCDD per kg body weight. There was a dose-related increase in mortality, both with respect to TCDD and the endotoxin. While the administration of 250 μg of endotoxin produced no mortality in the control group, as little as 10 μg of the endotoxin produced death in mice treated with 15 or 50 μg TCDD per kg. Similar increase in endotoxin sensitivity was reported when mice were treated with a single oral dose of 100 μg TCDD per kg and challenged with 20 μg of endotoxin. In all experiments, a TCDD dose-related decrease in body weight of animals and the weights of thymus and spleen was observed.

VII. EFFECT OF THYMOSIN TREATMENT ON TCDD-INDUCED IMMUNOSUPPRESSION

Since TCDD produces selective atrophy of the thymus, Vos et al.[12] studied the effect of thymosin on selected TCDD-induced immunosuppressive effects. Groups of newborn mice were injected subcutaneously with daily doses of 15 or 50 μg of calf thymosin for one week. The treatment was doubled during the second and tripled during the third week. Simultaneously, the thymosin-treated and control animals were exposed to TCDD via maternal treatment, 10 μg/kg, on days 1, 4, 8, 11, 15, and 18. Treatment of TCDD-exposed pups with thymosin significantly reduced their body weight and had no effect on thymus weights. Thymosin injections did not prevent the TCDD-induced reduction in the DNA synthesis of thymocytes when these cells were cultured in the presence of phytohemagglutinin, concanavalin A, or pokeweed mitogen. Serum zinc concentration was not influenced by the TCDD treatment suggesting that the immunosuppression was not mediated through zinc deficiency often associated with severe atrophy of lymphoid organs. The role of thymic hormones in TCDD-caused immunosuppression was hence not supported.

VIII. TCDD EFFECTS ON NONSPECIFIC PHAGOCYTOSIS BY SPLEEN OR PERIPHERAL MACROPHAGES

In the studies mentioned above, Vos and colleagues[12] reported the accumulation of *Listeria monocytogenes* in the spleen of TCDD-treated mice. The number of viable organisms in the spleen, 1 or 2 days after the intravenous injection of *L. monocytogenes* were not altered by 50 μg TCDD per kg, given once a week for 4 weeks. Similar treatment of mice with TCDD for 4 or 5 weeks, did not alter the number of macrophages harvested from the peritoneal cavity. The reduction of nitro-blue tetrazolium by the macrophages was not influenced by TCDD treatment. The results were interpreted to indicate that the treatment of animals with TCDD did not alter the macrophage function as proposed earlier by Thigpen et al.[17] The possible effect of TCDD on T cell-macrophage interactions was also not supported.

IX. TCDD-INDUCED IMMUNOSUPPRESSION IN RABBITS

Sharma et al.[14] have exposed adult male rabbits to 0.01, 0.1, 1, and 10 μg TCDD per kg orally for 8 weeks. After 4 and 6 weekly doses of TCDD, the animals were inoculated with a mixture of tetanus toxoid and Freund's Complete Adjuvant. Serum IgG levels were measured at various times during the experiment along with other hematological parameters, such as total and differential leukocyte counts and red cell concentration. The animals were tested for skin reactivity to tuberculin, 10 days after the respective antigen challenge. Serum antitetanus antibodies and the relative number of plasma cells in popliteal lymph nodes were evaluated. Three out of five rabbits given 10 μg TCDD per kg per week died during an 8-week experimental period. The weights of thymus, adrenals and popliteal lymph nodes were significantly depressed in animals treated with the highest dose of TCDD. A dose-related increase in liver weights was observed. Serum antitetanus titers showed a decrease at treatment levels starting from 0.1 μg/kg. Similarly, a significant decrease in the number of plasma cells in popliteal nodes was observed in groups treated with 1 or 10 μg TCDD per kg level. Skin reactivity to tuberculin was depressed at all TCDD dose levels, the suppression was related with increasing dose of TCDD. Serum IgG levels, however, were significantly increased at 0.01 and 0.1 μg TCDD per kg dose level, showing a decline at the higher levels of TCDD treatment with a significant decrease from the control values at the TCDD level of 10 μg/kg/week. The results were somewhat comparable to those reported in mice by Sharma and Gehring[13] using a similar protocol. It may be concluded that treatment of animals with TCDD produced effects on cell-mediated immune reactions at very low dose levels, whereas the effect on humoral immunity was observed at high dose levels. The effect on humoral immune responses may be an indirect one, produced by initial suppression of T cells involved in such mechanisms.

X. EFFECT OF TCDD EXPOSURE ON LYMPHOCYTE TRANSFORMATION IN CULTURES

Several studies have been reported where exposure of animals to TCDD has been shown to decrease the responsiveness of lymphocytes to various mitogens in culture. Results from selected studies have been summarized in Table 4. Many of the studies were conducted in conjunction with the experiments that are indicated earlier. Exposure of rats to various doses of TCDD, pre- and postnatally through maternal treatments, decreased the synthesis of DNA by splenic and thymic lymphocytes when cultured in the presence of phytohemagglutinin. The transformation of thymocytes in the presence of concanavalin A was not affected by the exposure of animals to TCDD, although a reduced size of thymus accounted for a depressed effect when the results were expressed on a whole organ basis.[16]

In the studies reported by Vos et al.,[16] the exposure of newborn mice via postnatal maternal treatment with TCDD decreased the mitogen-induced DNA synthesis in thymus cells when the lymphocytes were cultured in the presence of phytohemagglutinin, concanavalin A, or pokeweed mitogen. The decreased responsiveness of thymus cells to mitogens, together with the fact that there was a considerable depletion of cells in the thymus, suggested a strong immunosuppressive effect of TCDD treatment.

Splenic lymphocytes from mice treated with 0.01 to 10 μg TCDD per kg once a week for 2-8 weeks produced effects similar to those described above when the cells were cultured in the presence of phytohemagglutinin or pokeweed mitogen.[13] The effect was apparent within 2 weeks of treatment with the intensity of change declining after 8 weeks of treatment. One additional feature noted in the splenic cultures was that the cells from TCDD-exposed animals transformed at a higher rate than those in respective controls even in the absence of any mitogenic agent. The exact significance of spontaneous transformation of splenic lymphocytes in TCDD-treated animals was not well understood.

An effect similar to the one above was also observed in mice and rabbits when these animals were challenged with an appropriate antigen consisting of tetanus toxoid and Freund's Complete Adjuvant.[14] The increase in the spontaneous lymphocyte transformation from the spleen of treated animals was not so apparent; a decreased responsiveness to phytohemagglutinin-induced DNA synthesis was observed, particularly when the animals were treated with 10 μg TCDD per kg body weight for 8 weeks.

The effect of a single oral dose of 10 μg TCDD per kg in 2- and 6-month old mice was investigated. The results of splenic cell transformation are presented in Table 5. The effect of TCDD was less pronounced in older animals while the variability decreased as animals grew older. The stimulation indexes in splenic lymphocytes for phytohemagglutinin and pokeweed mitogen were significantly decreased in 6-month old animals.

Table 4
EFFECT OF TCDD EXPOSURE ON LYMPHOCYTE TRANSFORMATION

Species	Dose and schedule	Effects reported	Ref.
Rat	1 and 5 μg/kg × 3 to 5 doses	A decrease in splenic and thymus lymphocyte response to PHA; response to Con A/thymus decreased	16
Mice	10 μg/kg, twice weekly for 3 weeks to nursing dams starting day 1	Decreased response of thymus cells to PHA, PWM, and Con A, at 22 days of age	12
Mice	0.01—10 μg/kg weekly for 2—8 weeks	Dose-related decrease in PHA and PWM induced transformation at 2 and 4 weeks of exposure; no consistent effect observed at dose levels of ≥0.1 μg/kg after 2 weeks; A dose related increase in lymphocyte transformation without any mitogen seen at all times	13
Rabbits	0.01—10 μg weekly for 8 weeks, the animals challenged with tetanus toxoid	A decrease in PHA response at the highest dose; Increase in thymidine incorporation of unstimulated cultures at 1 μg/kg	14

Table 5
RESPONSE OF YOUNG VS. MATURE MICE SPLENIC LYMPHOCYTES IN SPLENIC CULTURES TO PHYTOHEMAGGLUTININ AND POKEWEED MITOGEN AFTER IN VIVO EXPOSURE TO TETRACHLORODIBENZO-*p*-DIOXIN[a]

Treatment group and age of mice at TCDD exposure	DPM/10[6] cells without mitogen	Stimulation index with	
		PHA	PWM
Control, 2-month	37,522 ± 12,965	1.2 ± 0.8	12.6 ± 10.4
TCDD treated, 2-month	339,234 ± 119,811[b]	0.5 ± 0.3	1.1 ± 0.5
Control, 6-month	3,501 ± 646	11.6 ± 2.6	8.0 ± 1.1
TCDD treated, 6-month	5,821 ± 1,718	5.2 ± 1.1[b]	4.5 ± 0.5[b]

[a] Animals were treated orally with a single dose of 10 μg TCDD per kg body weight and their spleens cultured 2 weeks after the treatment; Sharma, R. P., unpublished data; all values are mean ± SE.

[b] Significantly different from respective control at $p < 0.05$.

XI. EFFECT OF IN VITRO TCDD EXPOSURE ON LYMPHOCYTES

The influence of direct addition of TCDD to mouse-splenic cultures was reported by Sharma and Gehring.[13] TCDD decreased the unstimulated DNA synthesis in lymphocytes at concentrations as low as 10^{-9} *M*. The relative effect of phytomitogens, phytohemagglutinin, and pokeweed mitogen was also reduced in these cultures. TCDD, up to 10^{-4} *M* produced no effect on mitogen-induced lymphocyte stimulation indexes. It is possible that TCDD was cytotoxic to certain lymphocytes, whereas others were not affected and could be stimulated by a mitogenic stimulus.

Vos and Moore[17] have reported that the addition of TCDD up to 0.01 $\mu g/0.5\ m\ell$ in culture medium did not alter the DNA synthesis in mouse spleen or rat thymus cells, either with or without the presence of phytohemagglutinin or concanavalin A.

Luster and co-workers[18] exposed spleens from mice to TCDD in dimethylsulfoxide. DNA, RNA, and protein synthesis in spleens were inhibited at TCDD concentrations of 10^{-7} *M*. The ability of lymphocytes to bind with mitogens was not influenced by TCDD.

XII. REVERSAL OF IMMUNE EFFECTS IN TCDD-TREATED ANIMALS

Sharma et al.[19] reported that immunologic effects of a single dose of TCDD in mice were reversible during an 8-week period, while the hepatic lesions persisted. Mice were treated with a single oral dose of 10 μg TCDD per kg, and selected animals sacrificed at 2, 4, and 8 weeks after this dosing. The spontaneous increase of DNA synthesis in splenic cultures, and a decreased responsiveness of splenic lymphocytes to phytohemagglutinin and pokeweed mitogen was apparent at 2 weeks after the treatment. The effects persisted up to 4 weeks after the administration of TCDD but were not noticed when the spleens were obtained from animals at 8 weeks after the TCDD dosing. Even the lymphocyte-depletion in thymus and thymus weights showed a partial recovery at this period.

The depression of cell-mediated immune responses in rats exposed inutero or shortly after birth through maternal dosing with TCDD persisted up to 145 days of age.[18] The effects were less severe in newborn animals exposed postnatally only. The humoral responses in these animals were not affected and the helper T cell function was also not depressed.

XIII. EPIDEMIOLOGICAL CONSIDERATIONS

Because of the widespread existence of TCDD as a contaminant in various industrial products, particularly various chlorinated phenols, several epidemics caused by environmental exposures to this toxic chemical have occurred. In the environment TCDD is a very persistent compound, its half-life in soil being about 1 year.[20] Chlorinated dioxins are believed to be the causative agent of chick edema disease which produced a measurable loss in the poultry industry.[21] TCDD was identified in various fish and crustacean samples collected from South Vietnam after the herbicide 2,4,5-T was used in that country.[22]

Contamination of a farm in eastern Missouri by waste oils contaminated with TCDD caused deaths of many horses, birds, rodents, cats, dogs, and insects.[23] Although none of the animals were examined specifically for effects on immune organs, microscopic evaluation of spleens taken from horses during this episode indicated atrophy of this organ, and congestion and thickening of the capsule.

The most dramatic episode of environmental contamination by TCDD was illustrated by an industrial accident in Seveso, Italy in 1976.[24] The reactor involved in this accident was used for the manufacture of trichlorophenol for the ultimate production of herbicides. The contamination of the surrounding area after the explosion of the reactor resulted in the evacuation of the affected inhabitants from roughly 400 acres, with possible contamination of a much larger area. A large scale screening of children from this area resulted in a number of confirmed chloracne cases. The unfortunate accident provided a means for evaluating various immune functions in exposed individuals. However, preliminary reports have shown no definite effects on the immunologic parameters, except for a transient decrease of lymphocytes.[25]

XIV. CONCLUSIONS

This review indicates that TCDD is a potent immunosuppressant. The immune effects, however, were apparent at exposure levels that also produced other discernible pathological lesions, particularly in the liver and thymus. The exact mechanism of TCDD-induced immunosuppression is still unknown. It may be said that cell-mediated immunity functions are influenced by TCDD at much lower concentrations than those producing humoral effects. The latter may be affected indirectly via T cell mechanisms that are generally involved in recognition or other complex humoral pathways. All of the species of laboratory animals treated with TCDD show immunosuppression although no known effect of this kind in exposed people has been illustrated. In animals the effects appear to be reversible, the period of reversal depending on the half-life of TCDD in a given species. The toxicity and half-life of TCDD is largely species-dependent.

More information, particularly on the mechanism by which TCDD induces immunosuppression, needs to be known before its public health hazard can be accurately evaluated. This extremely toxic chemical provides a valuable tool for studying the cellular or molecular steps that lead to the modification of immune responses by environmental chemicals.[9]

REFERENCES

1. **Schwetz, B. A., Norris, J. M., Sparschu, G. L., Rowe, V. K., Gehring, P. J., Emerson, J. L., and Gerbig, C. G.**, Toxicology of chlorinated dibenzo-*p*-dioxins, *Environ. Health Perspect.*, 5, 87, 1973.
2. **Elvidge, D. A.**, The gas chromatographic determination of 2, 3,7,8-tetrachlorodibenzo-*p*-dioxin in 2,4,5-trichlorophenoxyacetic acid and 2,4,5-T esters and 2,4,5-trichlorophenol, *Analyst*, 96, 721, 1971.
3. **Woolson, E. A., Thomas, R. F., and Ensor, P. D. J**, Survey of polychlorodibenzo-*p*-dioxin content in selected pesticides, *J. Agric. Food Chem.*, 20, 351, 1972.
4. **Gupta, B. N., Vos, J. G., Moore, J. A., Zinkl, J. G., and Bullock, B. C.**, Pathologic effects of 2,3,7,8-tetrachlorodibenzo-*p*-dioxin in laboratory animals, *Environ. Health Perspect.*, 5, 125, 1973.
5. **Buu-Hoi, N. P., Chanh, P. H., Sesque, G., Azum-Gelade, M. C., and Saint-Ruf, G.**, Organs as targets of dioxin (2,3,7,8-tetrachlorodibenzo-*p*--dioxin) intoxication, *Naturwissenschaften*, 59, 174, 1972.
6. **Vos, J. G., Moore, J. A., and Zinkl, J. G.**, Effect of 2,3,7,8-tetrachlorodibenzo-*p*-dioxin on the immune system of laboratory animals, *Environ. Health Perspect.*, 5, 149, 1973.
7. **Zinkl, J. G., Vos, J. G., Moore, J. A., and Gupta, B. N.**, Hematologic and clinical chemistry effects of 2,3,7,8-tetrachlorodibenzo-*p*-dioxin in laboratory animals, *Environ. Health Perspect.*, 5, 111, 1973.
8. **Courtney, K. D. and Moore, J. A.**, Teratology studies with 2,4,5-trichlorophenoxyacetic acid and 2,3,7,8-tetrachlorodibenzo-*p*-dioxin, *Toxicol. Appl. Pharmacol.*, 20, 396, 1971.
9. **Poland, A. and Kende, A.**, 2,3,7,8-tetrachlorodibenzo-*p*-dioxin: environmental contaminant and molecular probe., *Fed. Proc. Fed. Am. Soc. Exp. Bio.*, 35, 2404, 1976.
10. **Vos, J. G., Moore, J. A., and Zinkl, J. G.**, Toxicity of 2,3,7,8-tetrachlorodibenzo-*p*-dioxin (TCDD) in C57Bl/6 mice, *Toxicol. Appl. Pharmacol.*, 29, 229, 1974.
11. **Kociba, R. J., Keeler, P. A., Park, C. N., and Gehring, P. J.**, 2,3,7,8-tetrachlorodibenzo-*p*-dioxin (TCDD): results of a 13-week oral toxicity study in rats, *Toxicol. Appl. Pharmacol.*, 35, 553, 1975.
12. **Vos, J. G., Kreeftenberg, J. G., Engel, H. W. B., Minderhoud, A., and Van Noorle Jansen, L. M.**, Studies on 2,3,7,8-tetrachlorodibenzo-*p*-dioxin induced immune suppression and decreased resistance to infection: endotoxin hypersensitivity, serum zinc concentrations and effect of thymosin treatment, *Toxicology*, 9, 75, 1978.

13. **Sharma, R. P. and Gehring, P. J.,** Effects of 2,3,7,8-tetrachlorodibenzo-*p*-dioxin (TCDD) on splenic lymphocyte transformation in mice after single and repeated exposures, *Ann. N.Y. Acad. Sci.* 320, 487, 1979.
14. **Sharma, R. P., Kociba, R. J., and Gehring, P. J.** Immontoxicologic effects of 2,3,7,8-tetrachlorodibenzo-*p*-dioxin (TCDD) in mice and rabbits, *J. Environ. Pathol. Toxicol.*, In press.
15. **McConnell, E. E., Moore, J. A., and Dalgard, D. W.,** Toxicity of 2,3,7,8-tetrachlorodibenzo-*p*-dioxin in rhesus monkeys *Macaca mulatta* following a single oral dose, *Toxicol. Appl. Pharmacol.*, 43, 175, 1978.
16. **Vos, J. G. and Moore, J. A.,** Suppression of cellular immunity in rats and mice by maternal treatment with 2,3,7,8-tetrachlorodibenzo-*p*-dioxin, *Int. Arch. Allergy*, 47, 777, 1974.
17. **Thigpen, J. E., Faith, R. E., McConnell, E. E., and Moore, J. A.,** Increased susceptibility to bacterial infection as a sequela of exposure to an environmental contaminant 2,3,7,8-tetrachlorodibenzo-*p*-dioxin (TCDD), *Infect. Immun.*, 12, 1319, 1975.
18. **Luster, M. I., Faith, R. E., and Clark, G.,** Laboratory studies on immune effects of halogenated aromatics, *Ann. N.Y. Acad. Sci.*, 320, 473, 1979.
19. **Sharma, R. P., Kociba, R. J., and Gehring, P. J.,** Reversal of immunologic and toxicologic effects of a single exposure of 2,3,7,8-tetrachlorodibenzo-*p*-dioxin in mice, Trace substances in *Environ. Health*, 12, 473, 1979.
20. **Kearney, P. C., Woolson, E. A., and Ellinpton, C. P.,** Persistence and metabolism of chlorodioxins in soils, *Environ. Sci. Technol.*, 6, 1017, 1972.
21. **Cantrell, J. S., Webb, N. C., and Mabis, J. J.,** Identification and crystal structure of a hydropericardium producing factor: 1,2,3,7,8,9-hexachlorodibenzo-*p*-dioxin, *Acta Cryst., allogr. Sect. B.*, 25, 150, 1969.
22. **Baughman, R., and Meselson, M.,** An analytical method for detecting TCDD (dioxin) levels of TCDD in samples from Vietnam, *Environ. Health Perspect*, 5, 27, 1973.
23. **Kimbrough, R. D. Carter, C. D., Liddle, J. A., Cline, R. E., and Phillips, P. E.,** Epidemiology and pathology of a tetrachlorodibenzo-*p*-dioxin poisoning episode, *Arch. Environ. Health*. 32, 77, 1977.
24. **Walsh, J., Seveso:** The question persists where dioxin created a wasteland, *Science*, 197, 1064, 1977.
25. **Reggiani, G.,** Medical problems raised by the TCDD contamination in Seveso, Italy, *Arch. Toxicol.*, 40, 161, 1978.

Chapter 10

IMMUNOTOXICITY OF ALKYLTIN COMPOUNDS*

Willem Seinen

TABLE OF CONTENTS

* This work was supported in part by the Dutch Cancer Foundation. (K.W.F.). Grant nr. UKC-PFT 78-3.

I. INTRODUCTION

A. Use of Organotin Compounds

Tin and its alloys played an important part in man's emergence from the Stone Age and have since made valuable contributions to man's economy.[1] Organotin compounds, already developed by Löwig[2] in 1852 and Frankland[3] in 1853, received industrial application especially during the past 25 years. The first organotin compound patented[4] was a tetraalkyltin compound used as a stabilizer of chlorinated transformer oils. The original development of organotin stabilizers for vinyl plastics was by Ingve[5] and since that time the commercial uses of organotins have developed rapidly. Today there are three main areas of application: (1) as heat stabilizers, especially for the stabilization of polyvinyl chloride plastics, (2) as biocidal compounds for wood, paper, and textile preservation, as an agricultural fungicide, miticide, and acaricide, and as a component of antifouling paints, and (3) as catalytic agents in a variety of industrial processes.[6,7,8] Although exact production data are not available, the estimated organotin production is more than 25,000 tons a year.[8,9]

B. Entry of Organotin Compounds Into Biological Systems

The entry of organotins into biological systems may have profound implications for human and environmental health. Direct introduction into man may occur by the migration of stabilizers from plastic into food, beverages, and drinking water, or from plastic medical devices into body fluids. Introduction into the environment occurs by the agricultural use of organotin compounds and also by leaching from plastic disposables which accounts for approximately 5% of the total solid waste disposal.[10] Although organotins are subject to chemical, microbial, and physical degradation to nontoxic inorganic tin, as is claimed by Van der Kerk,[11] information about the degradation rate and distribution of the various organotin compounds in the environment is rather scanty or even lacking. Therefore, the possibility of environmental effects of organotin pollution may exist. Also there are many possibilities for the entry of organotins from the environment into man. Concentration mechanisms through the food chain as known from halogenated aromatic hydrocarbons are not very likely, but can not be excluded yet.

C. General Toxicity of Organotin Compounds

Organotin compounds have received more attention for their biological effects than organic compounds of any other metal, with the possible exception of organomercurials. One of the many reasons for the broad interest in the toxicology of organotins is the "Stalinon affair", a French tragedy caused by the treatment of furuncles and other staphlococcal skin infections with a preparation called "Stalinon".[12] The main active components of this preparation were diethyltindiiodide and linoleic acid, but a certain batch also contained impurities of mono- and triethyltin. Two hundred and seventeen people are known to have been poisoned by the "Stalinon" preparation and one hundred of these people died.[13] Neurological symptoms were observed in all of the afflicted patients surveyed by Alajonanine et al.[13] In the four cases examined histologically,[14] a marked interstitial edema of the white matter of the brain was noted, which is characteristic for a triethyltin intoxication.[15] Following the Stalinon affair, the toxicity of organotin compounds has been widely studied. It has been reviewed extensively by Barnes and Stoner[12] and more recently by Piver.[10]

The toxicity of alkyltin compounds is determined by the nature of the organic group bound to tin, whereas the nature of the anionic group is only of secondary importance. Distinction must be noted between the biological activity of tetra-, tri-, di-, and monoalkyltins. The trialkyltin compounds, especially triethyl and trimethyltins, affect the central nervous system, producing cerebral edema. The oral toxicity of trialkyltins progressively diminish from tri-n-propyl to tri-n-hexyltin with tri-n-octyltin being nontoxic.[17] Tetraalkyltin compounds act toxicologically similar to trialkyltins by virtue of their enzymatic conversion by liver microsomal enzymes to trialkyltins.[18] The toxicity of monoalkyltin compounds is low.[19] The dialkyltin compounds from methyl to hexyl induce bile duct lesions[20] in rats and mice, but not in rabbits or guinea pigs. The lower homologues in the dialkyltin series also cause skin irritation. The higher homologues — octyl or above — seemed to be very less toxic by oral administration.[17] Recently, effects on the immune system have been discovered as the most sensitive criteria of toxicity of certain organotin compounds.[22-27]

Although immunology had a more expansive growth than any other discipline in biomedical research during the last decade, the knowledge about the immune system is rarely incorporated in the evaluation of the toxicity of chemicals including organotins. For example, in the appraisals for toxicity testing of the Food and Drug Administration[28] and the World Health Organization,[29,30] a procedure for the evaluation on effects on the immune system are lacking. This is probably one of the reasons why the immunotoxicity of organotin compounds were overlooked. At the moment the number of chemicals that are known to induce immune alterations is growing, as is the interest in the field of immunotoxicology as shown in a recent review.[31] Now the possibility of immune alterations by chemicals is also recognized by the expert committee on food additives of the Dutch Voedingsraad.[32]

II. EFFECTS OF DIALKYLTIN COMPOUNDS ON LYMPHOID ORGANS

In order to reinvestigate the general toxicity of di-n-octyltindichloride (DOTC) a six-week toxicity study was performed with rats fed dietary levels of 0, 50, or 150 ppm (mg/kg) DOTC.[22] At 150 ppm a slight but significant growth retardation associated with a slightly decreased food efficiency was noted. Serum alkaline phosphatase (AP) activity was significantly increased both at 50 and 150 ppm, which was accompanied by increased AP activities in kidney and liver homogenates. Treatment-related histopathological changes were only observed in lymphoid organs. A dose-dependent depletion of lymphocytes was seen in thymus (Figures 1—3) and thymus-dependent areas of spleen and peripheral lymph nodes. Feeding of rats 50 or 150 ppm DOTC for 4 weeks reduced thymus weight by 52 and 84%, respectively (Figure 4). The number and viability of cells that could be isolated from DOTC-fed rats declined rapidly and in a dose-related fashion. Four weeks feeding 50 and 150 ppm DOTC reduced the number of thymocytes by 67 and 94%, respectively. Also the number and viability of cells isolated from the spleen were decreased by DOTC feeding, but this effect was less pronounced as on thymus. In contrast, no effect was found on cell counts and viability of bone marrow cells.[22] The effect of dialkyltin compounds on bone marrow is further analysed in mice intravenously dosed with di-n-butyltindichloride (DBTC), a compound with effects on lymphoid tissues similar to those observed with DOTC. Three days after treatment with 10 mg DBTC/kg body weight, the number of thymocytes was decreased by 71%, whereas the number of bone marrow cells was not affected (Table 1). As compared to the controls, the DNA synthesis of thymocytes, as measured by the incorporation of ^{3}H-thymidine into DNA, was markedly decreased whereas the ^{3}H-thymidine incorporation of bone marrow cells was unaffected. Also, there was no effect of DBTC treatment on bone marrow stem cells as measured with the spleen colony assay technique of Till and McCullouch.[33] The numbers of 10-day spleen colonies produced in lethally irradiated recipient mice injected with bone marrow cells of donor mice treated 1 or 3 days before cell transplantation with 0 or 10 mg DBTC/kg intravenously, were essentially the same.[26]

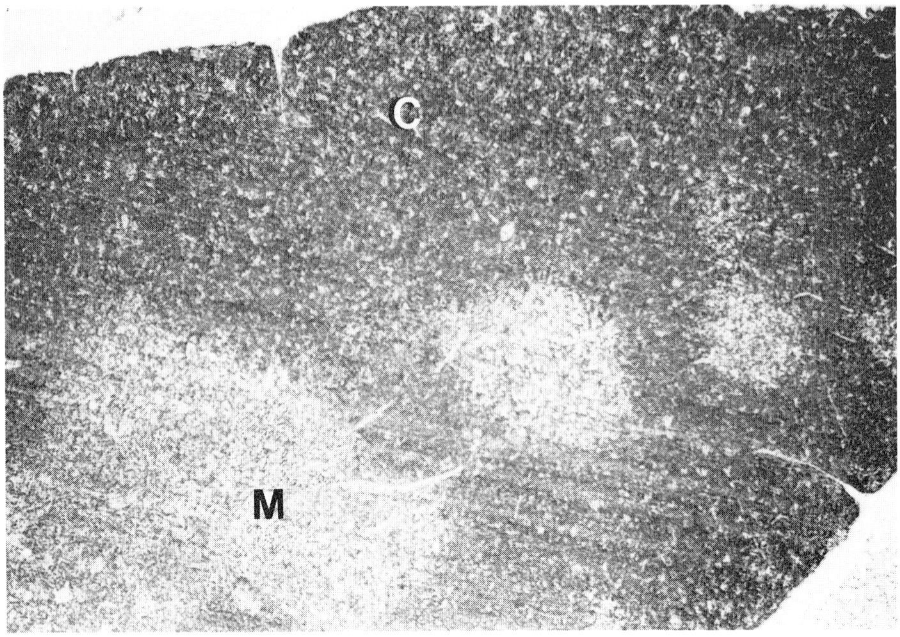

FIGURE 1. Part of a thymus from a control rats showing a well-developed cortex (C) and medulla (M). Hematoxylin and eosin; magnification × 60.

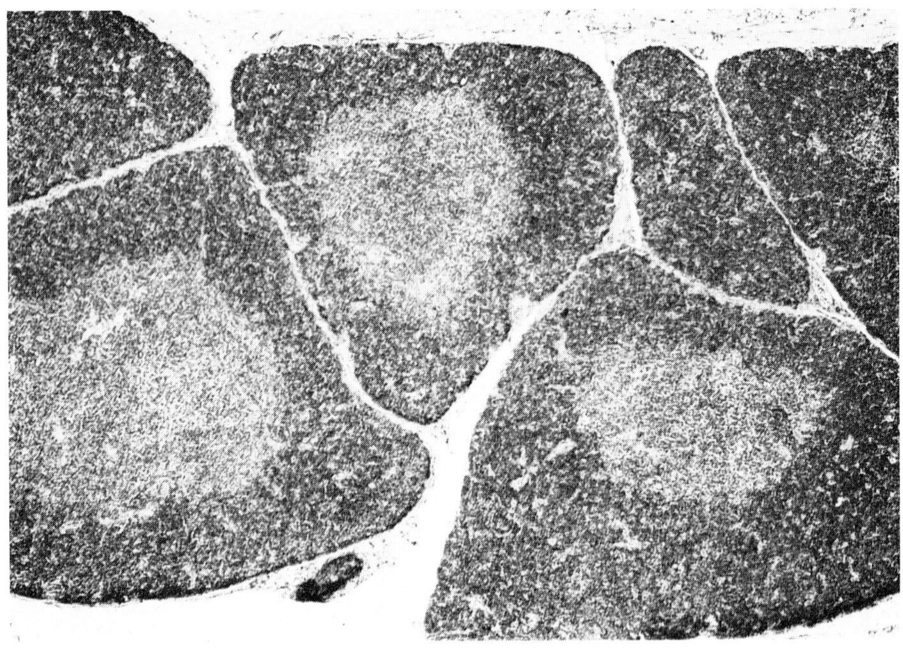

FIGURE 2. Part of a thymus from a rat treated with 50 ppm DOTC for 6 weeks. Note the atrophy of the thymic cortex. Hematoxylin and eosin; magnification × 60.

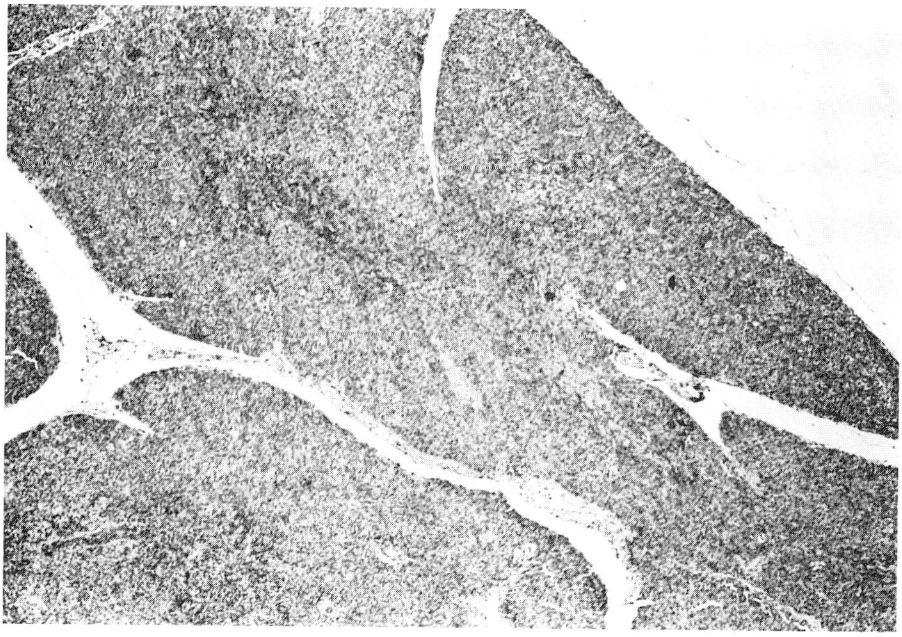

FIGURE 3. Part of a thymus from a rat fed 150 ppm DOTC for 6 weeks showing complete lymphocyte depletion of the cortex. At this magnification, no distinction can be made between cortex and medulla. Hematoxylin and eosin; magnification × 60.

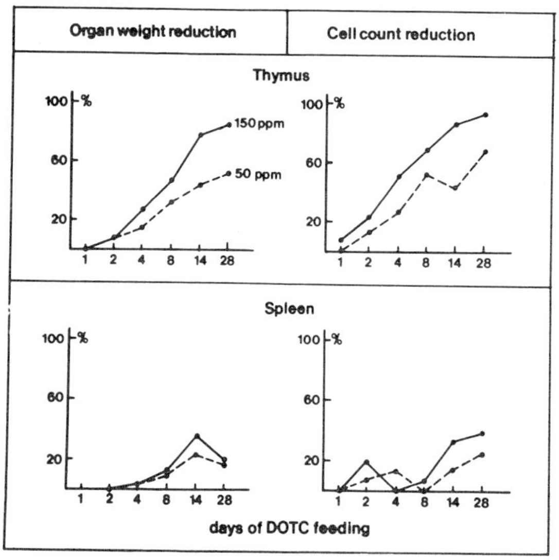

FIGURE 4. Reduction of weight and total necleated cell count of thymus and spleen from rats fed 0, 50, or 150 ppm DOTC for 1, 2, 4, 8, 14, and 28 days. Results are given in percentages and are means of four animals.

Table 1
TOTAL NUMBER AND DNA-REPLICATION OF THYMUS AND BONE MARROW CELLS OF DBTC-TREATED MICE[a]

I.V. dose of DBTC (mg/kg)	Total cell count (× 10^6)		^{3}H-thymidine incorporation[b] (cpm)	
	Thymus	Bone marrow	Thymus	Bone marrow
0	408 ± 23	320 ± 40	11,550 ± 424	23,780 ± 1,168
10	118 ± 18[c]	293 ± 15	3,366 ± 487[c]	26,470 ± 2,617

[a] Mean values ± SEM. Groups of 10 balb/c mice were intravenously dosed with DBTC and killed 3 days after injection. Bone marrow cells were obtained by flushing medium through the femoral and tibial marrow cavity of both hind legs. A suspension of isolated cells was prepared by passing through a nylon sieve (220 μm pore diameter).
[b] Cells were cultured in microtiter plates (4 × 10^5 cells/well) in the presence of 0.25 μ Ci ^{3}H-thymidine (SA 0.5 Ci/mMol) for 24 hr.
[c] $p < 0.001$.

Since lymphocytotoxicity is observed in dialkyltin treated rats at concentrations that do not induce a generalized toxicity nor a myelotoxicity, it was concluded that DBTC and DOTC exert a selective cytotoxic effect on lymphocytes in thymus and thymus-dependent areas of peripheral lymphoid organs.

A stress-related release of glucocorticosteroids as in intermediate was not observed in adrenalectomized rats exposed to DOTC, thus suggesting that the effects were directly on the lymphoid system. Thymus weights of adrenalectomized rats was as severely decreased by DOTC treatment as the thymus weight of the sham-operated control animals.[22] A direct effect on the lymphoid system is further supported by the cytotoxic effect of dialkyltin compounds on thymocytes in vitro.[23,25]

In order to study the long-lasting effect of DOTC, rats were fed diets containing 0 or 150 ppm for 4 weeks and after that period returned to stock diet to investigate the reversibility of DOTC-induced thymus involution.[23] Within 16 days of rehabilitation thymus weights returned to control values, which is suggestive of a short half-life of DOTC.

Comparative short-term toxicity studies were carried out with rats to determine the relationship between the chemical structure of various alkyltin compounds and their thymolytic effects.[23] These feeding studies revealed that not only DOTC and DBTC, but also, although to lesser extent, di-n-propyltindichloride (DPTC) and diethyltindichloride (DETC) reduced the weight of the thymus, spleen, and popliteal lymph node in a dose-dependent fashion. It was associated with a depletion of lymphocytes in the cortex of the thymus and the thymus-dependent lymphoid areas of the peripheral lymphoid organs. In contrast, dimethyltindichloride, di-n-dodecyltindibromide, and di-n-octadecyltindibromide did not cause atrophy of lymphoid organs.

Of the trialkyltins, tri-n-butyltindichloride caused thymus atrophy comparable to di-n-butyltindichloride, whereas trimethyl, triethyl and tri-n-octyltinchloride did not induce thymus atrophy. Mono-n-octyltintrichloride and tetra-n-octyltin did not cause any organ change at feeding levels up to 150 ppm.

Since the degree of dialkyltin-induced thymus atrophy is strongly related to the length of the alkyl chain (Figure 5), it is probably related to the water:lipid partition of the homologues. Upon intravenous administration of the various dialkyltin compounds a similar structure-activity relationship regarding thymus atrophy was found, as upon their oral administration.[23] Single, as well as repeated, i.v. injections of 1 or 2 mg DBTC or

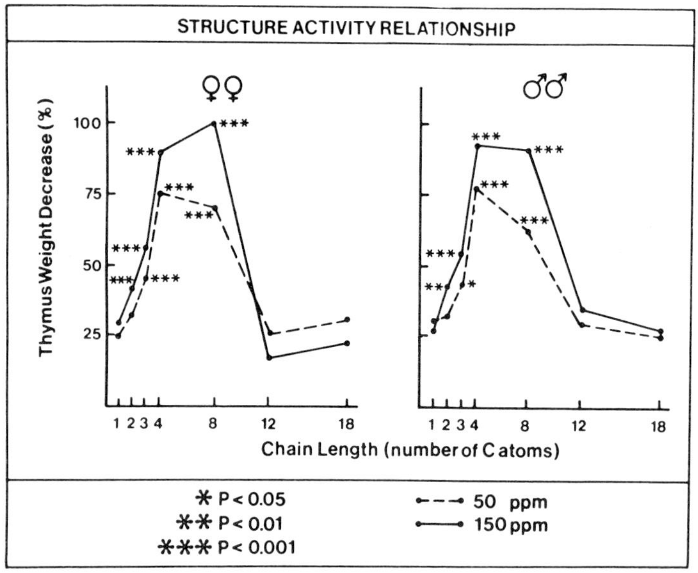

FIGURE 5. Relationship between length of the alkyl chain of dialkyltin compounds and its effect on thymus weight determined in groups of ten male and ten female rats fed various dialkyltin compounds at 0, 50, or 150 ppm for 2 weeks.

DOTC/kg body weight induced thymus atrophy without affecting the growth of the animals or the weights and histology of liver and kidney.

Comparative feeding studies in different animal species showed that DOTC and DBTC did not induce a selective lymphoid atrophy in mice, guinea pigs, and Japanese quail.[23]

III. IN VITRO CYTOTOXICITY STUDIES WITH DBTC AND DOTC

Dialkyltin compounds are extremely cytotoxic in vitro.[24,25] In suspension cultures of rat thymocytes, cell survival decreased in direct proportion to the DBTC or DOTC concentration in the nutrient medium. A concentration as low as 0.5 μg DBTC/mℓ medium markedly decreased the thymocyte survival within 24 hr of incubation. In contrast, the number and viability of rat bone marrow cells was not reduced by DOTC or DBTC in concentrations up to 50 μg/mℓ medium, when cultured for periods up to 40 hr under the same conditions as rat thymocytes. These data demonstrate a selective cytotoxicity of these organotin compounds in vitro.

Cytotoxicity of DBTC and DOTC was also shown in a graft vs. host (GVH) experiment in which thymus and peripheral lymph node cells from WAG rats were incubated in vitro for 4 hr with various concentrations of the organotin compounds and injected into the hind feet of (WAG $\times$ B) F_1 recipients. The increase of popliteal lymph node (PLN) weight in the F_1 animals is a measure of the GVH reactivity of the inoculated cell suspension.[38] The results of this experiment are given in Table 2. The popliteal lymph node weights of the recipient animals inoculated with thymus and PLN cells incubated with 10 μg DBTC or 50 μg DOTC/mℓ medium approached the popliteal lymph node weight of the uninjected control feet. Therefore, it was concluded that this treatment completely abolished GVH-inducing ability of the lymphocytes. A concentration of 0.1 μg DBTC or 0.5 μg DOTC/mℓ medium did not reduce the GVH reactivity of thymus and PLN cells (Figure 6).

Table 2
THE IN VITRO EFFECTS OF VARIOUS CONCENTRATIONS OF DBTC AND DOTC ON THE GRAFT VS. HOST REACTIVITY OF THYMUS AND PERIPHERAL LYMPH NODE (PLN) CELLS[a]

Conc. of organotin compound (μg/mℓ)	Organ and number of cells inoculated	Popliteal lymph node weights[b] (mg)
DOTC, 0 (control) Thymus,	0	5.0 ± 0.5
	2 × 10⁷	25.3 ± 7.3
	4 × 10⁷	33.5 ± 10.3
	8 × 10⁷	59.3 ± 11.3
0.5	2 × 10⁷	17.8 ± 5.0
	4 × 10⁷	36.7 ± 8.6
	8 × 10⁷	51.0 ± 7.9
50	2 × 10⁷	6.0 ± 1.5[c]
	4 × 10⁷	7.4 ± 3.4[c]
	8 × 10⁷	7.5 ± 1.7[c]
DOTC, 0 PLN,	0	4.8 ± 0.7
	0.33 × 10⁶	7.0 ± 2.8
	1 × 10⁶	19.8 ± 5.5
	3 × 10⁶	47.9 ± 12.0
±0.5	0.33 × 10⁶	6.8 ± 2.0
	1 × 10⁶	18.9 ± 7.4
	3 × 10⁶	40.6 ± 9.7
50	0.33 × 10⁶	5.5 ± 0.4
	1 × 10⁶	6.3 ± 0.3[c]
	3 × 10⁶	5.3 ± 0.3[c]
DBTC, 0 (control) Thymus,	0	5.2 ± 1.4
	2 × 10⁷	33.8 ± 9.5
	4 × 10⁷	32.8 ± 9.0
	8 × 10⁷	71.1 ± 6.3
0.1	2 × 10⁷	26.3 ± 9.0
	4 × 10⁷	34.6 ± 12.0
	8 × 10⁷	63.5 ± 8.7
10	2 × 10⁷	5.7 ± 1.3[c]
	4 × 10⁷	6.4 ± 0.8[c]
	8 × 10⁷	7.5 ± 1.7[c]
DBTC, 0 PLN,	0.33 × 10⁶	14.2 ± 6.8
	1 × 10⁶	18.1 ± 6.8
	3 × 10⁶	50.0 ± 7.2
0.1	1 × 10⁶	19.4 ± 7.2
	3 × 10⁶	45.7 ± 5.9
10	0.33 × 10⁶	5.4 ± 1.9[c]
	1 × 10⁶	5.1 ± 1.1[c]
	3 × 10⁶	5.4 ± 0.8[c]

[a] Cells were cultured for 4 hr in a CO_2-incubator in RPMI-1640 medium with 0, 0.1 or 10μg DBTC/mℓ or 0 , 0.5, or 50μ DOTC/mℓ at a concentration of 1 × 10^8 cell/mℓ.

[b] Mean values ± SD of 8 popliteal lymph nodes of (WAG × B) F_1 recipient animals inoculated with various numbers of organotin exposed lymphocytes of WAG rats.

[c] $p < 0.001$.

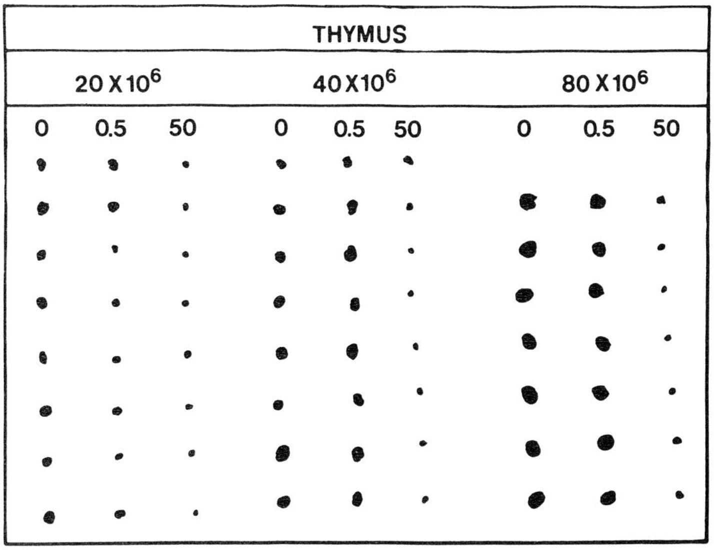

FIGURE 6. Popliteal lymph nodes of WAG × B hybrid rats, 7 days after injection with 20, 40, or 80 million WAG thymocytes incubated with 0, 0.5, or 50 μg DOTC/mℓ for 4 hr.

In cell viability tests[24] a marked difference in organotin sensitivity was noted between thymocytes from various species. In mouse and guinea pig thymocytes cultured for 24 hr in the presence of 50 μg DBTC/mℓ medium no effect was found on the number and viability of these cells. Also, the viability of human thymocytes was not distinctly decreased, but these cells aggregated in a dose-dependent fashion in the presence of 0.5 μg and more DBTC or DOTC per mℓ medium.[25] Cell agglutination could be prevented when human thymocytes were cultured at low concentrations in a shaking waterbath. But, the ability of these cells to form E-rosettes was rapidly reduced in direct proportion to the concentration of the organotin compounds in the incubation medium. Concentrations as low as 0.02 μg DBTC/mℓ and 0.5 μg DOTC/mℓ already decreased the formation of E rosettes (Figure 7).

A direct cytotoxicity of dialkyltin compounds on lymphocytes was also demonstrated in ^{3}H-thymidine incorporation studies.[26] DNA-synthesis of rat as well as human thymocytes was already inhibited at concentrations as low as 0.02 μg DBTC or 0.1 μg DOTC/mℓ medium. Other dialkyltin compounds also induced inhibition of DNA-replication and no distinct differences in antiproliferative activity of the various dialkyltins were observed in vitro. Therefore, the differences in lymphocytotoxicity observed after in vivo treatment of rats, between the water soluble and water insoluble dialkyltins can not be explained by differences in in vitro activity of these compounds.

Not only was the incorporation of ^{3}H-thymidine of rat and human thymocytes inhibited at very low dialkyltin concentrations, but also rat bone marrow cells and mouse thymus and bone marrow cells and various tumor cells were also affected by the in vitro exposure to DBTC and DOTC, though mostly at some higher concentrations (Figure 8).

From these incorporation studies it appears that while the dialkyltins are extremely cytotoxic in vitro, they do not display selectivity regarding the origin of the cells. Therefore, it is concluded that the selective effects on the lymphoid system seen upon in vivo exposure to DBTC and DOTC are not related to differences between various cells in the in vitro effects of organotin compounds upon DNA-replication. Possibly the selectivity

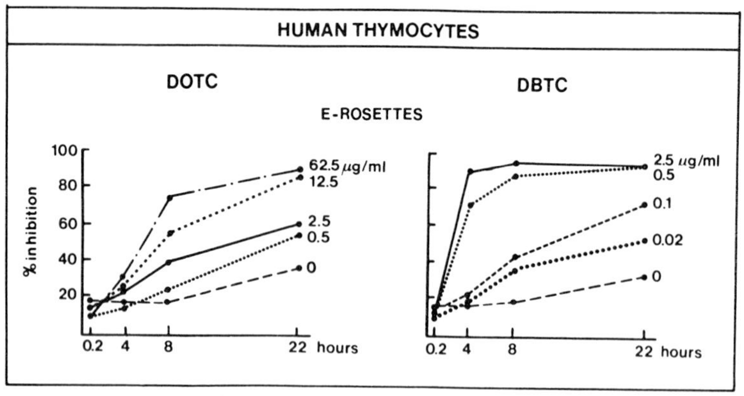

FIGURE 7. The in vitro effect of various concentrations of DBTC and DOTC upon the E-rosette formation. Three hundred thousand thymocytes were cultured in a total volume of 1 mℓ medium in polystyrene culture tubes incubated with various concentrations of the organotin compounds in a shaking waterbath. For the rosette formation, 1×10^7 SRBC were added to the cultures, after which the cells were centrifuged and the cell pellet was incubated at room temperature for 1 hr. Rosettes were defined microscopically by the agglutination of three or more SRBC around a nucleated cell. The decline of rosette forming cells in triplicate cultures is given in percentages.

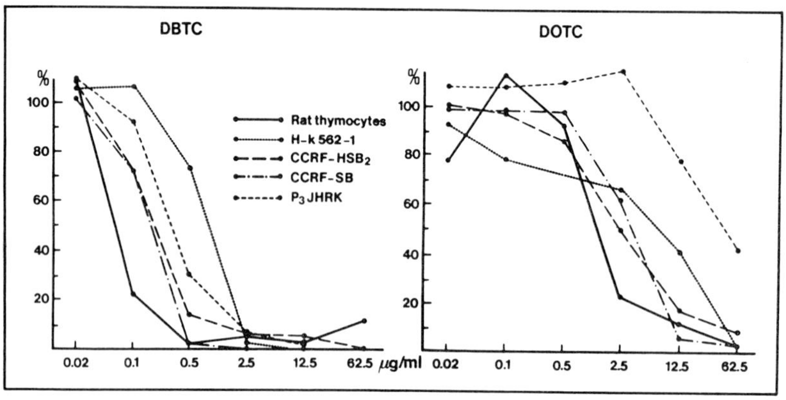

FIGURE 8. The in vitro effect of different concentrations of DBTC and DOTC upon ^{3}H-thymidine incorporation of rat thymocytes and various human lymphoid cell lines. Cells were cultured in triplicate during 72 hr and ^{3}H-thymidine was present during the last 24 hr of the culture period. Results are expressed as the mean percentages of the ^{3}H-thymidine incorporation of control cultures.

of action is related to the pharmacodynamic behavior of the dialkyltins in the body, a question which is under investigation at the moment.

IV. IMMUNE FUNCTION STUDIES WITH DBTC AND DOTC

Since the thymus and thymus-dependent lymphocytes play a central role in the immune system, an organotin-induced decrease of cells in thymus and thymus-dependent areas of peripheral lymphoid organs will result in an impairment of the immune system, and consequently in a decreased resistance against bacterial infections. From infection studies with *Listeria monocytogenes*, a T-cell-dependent phenomenon,[34] it appeared that DBTC and DOTC markedly increased the susceptibility of rats to this infection (Table 3). Four out of six animals fed 150 ppm DOTC for 4 weeks from weaning and all animals fed 150 ppm DBTC died from an i.v. injection with 0.5×10^6 *Listeria* organisms, whereas the control and 50 ppm fed animals all remained alive.

The resistance against a *Salmonella dublin* strain was also decreased by DBTC and DOTC, an effect possibly related to an increased susceptibility to *S. dublin* endotoxin since these organotin compounds are known to induce an increase of *Escherichia coli* lipopolysaccharide (LPS) sensitivity in rats (Table 4). After i.v. injections of 100, 300, and 900 μg *E. coli* LPS, 2, 4, and 5 rats died, respectively, at 150 ppm DOTC for 4-weeks 2, 4, and 5 rats died for 4-weeks from weaning, whereas 900 μg endotoxin did not induce lethality in the control animals. In the 50 ppm DOTC group lethality occurred in only two out of five animals injected with 900 μg of the endotoxin batch. Comparable results were obtained with DBTC-fed rats (Table 4). From the remaining animals injected with 100 μg LPS bloodserum was sampled 7 and 10 days after injection for the determination of the antibody titer against *E. coli* LPS. These titers were essentially the same in the DOTC- and DBTC-treated animals as well as in the controls (Table 5). It was also shown previously[24] that DBTC did not reduce the antibody production against the thymus-independent antigen LPS.

The inhibition of the thymus-dependent humoral immunity was shown by a reduction of plaque-forming cell numbers in the spleen as well as by a reduction of the hemagglutinin and hemolysin titers against sheep red blood cells in the serum of DBTC- and DOTC-exposed rats.[24] From other immune function studies, summarized in Table 6, it also appeared that all immune reactions in which T-lymphocytes participate are compromised in DBTC- or DOTC-exposed rats. A dose-related suppression of cell mediated immunity occurred in such manifestations as tuberculin hypersensitivity,[24] skin graft rejection,[24] graft vs. host reactivity and mitogen responsiveness.[25] The effect of postnatal treatment of rats with DOTC on the blast transformation of lymphocytes upon stimulation by the T-cell mitogens phytohemagglutinin (PHA) and concanavalin A (Con A) and the B-cell mitogen *E. coli* lipoploysaccharide (LPS) is shown in Figure 9. The mitogenic response of thymocytes, spleen cells, and peripheral lymph node cells to PHA and Con A was dose-relatedly decreased. Also the number of cells in the lymphoid organs was severely decreased (Figure 10). The thymus contained only 9 and 3%, respectively, of the number of thymocytes of control animals after postnatal treatment with 5 and 15 mg DOTC/kg. So, the mitogenic response to PHA and Con A calculated for the whole organs was dramatically decreased (Table 7).

In contrast, the ^{3}H-thymidine incorporation of spleen cells upon *E. coli* LPS stimulation was not impaired by the DOTC treatment. This supports the idea that dialkyltins suppress various subpopulations of T-lymphocytes without affecting B-cells. This selectivity may be explained by the selective depletion of lymphocytes in thymus and thymus-dependent lymphoid areas in the peripheral lymphoid organs of dialkyltin-exposed rats.

Macrophages do not seem to be compromised by organotin compounds since blood monocyte numbers and the phagocytizing capacity as measured by the clearance of carbon particles[24] were the same in treated and control animals. Therefore, it is concluded that DBTC and DOTC induce immune suppression in rats by a selective inhibition of T-lymphocyte activity.

The immunotoxicity of DBTC and DOTC was most pronounced in animals exposed to the chemicals during the developmental phase of the lymphoid system.[24,25] When rats were dosed by gavage with 5 mg DBTC/kg three times a week from day 2 after birth, growth stunting and mortality occurred without major pathology except for severe atrophy of lymphoid organs. Mortality also occurred in litters from rats kept on a 150 ppm

Table 3

RESISTANCE TO A *LISTERIA MONOCYTOGENES* INFECTION OF DBTC- OR DOTC-TREATED RATS[a]

Dietary Concentration (ppm)	Incidence of mortality[b]		
	0.5×10^6	1.5×10^6	4.5×10^6
DOTC			
0	0/6	5/6	6/6
50	0/6	6/6	6/6
150	4/6	6/6	6/6
DBTC			
0	0/6	4/6	6/6
50	0/6	4/6	6/6
150	6/6	6/6	6/6

[a] Rats were kept on diets with 0 , 50, or 150 ppm DBTC or DOTC for 4 weeks from weaning.

[b] Mortality was scored during ten days after an intravenous injection with the indicated number *Listeria monocytogenes* organisms.

Table 4

ESCHERICHIA COLI ENDOTOXIN SUSCEPTIBILITY OF DOTC-TREATED RATS[b]

Dietary concentration (ppm)	Incidence of mortality[b]		
	100μg LPS	300μg LPS	900μg LPS
DOTC			
0	0/5	0/5	0/5
50	0/5	0/5	2/5
150	2/5	4/5	5/5
DBTC			
0	0/5	0/5	0/5
50	0/5	1/5	3/5
150	0/5	2/5	5/5

[a] Rats were kept on diets with 0 , 50, or 150 ppm DOTC or DBTC for 4 weeks from weaning.

[b] Intravenous injection with endotoxin (lipopolysaccharide *E. coli* 0 127:B8). Mortality scored after 48 hr.

DOTC diet during pregnancy. Eighty percent of the pups died before the age of one month with morphological changes in the lymphoid organs which are suggestive of a runting syndrome as first described by Miller[35] in neonatal thymectomized mice. It is also observed in rats pups exposed perinatally by maternal treatment with busulfan[36] and 2,3,7,8-tetrachlorodibenzo-*p*-dioxin (TCDD).[37]

Table 5
HEMAGGLUTINATING ANTIBODY RESPONSE AGAINST *ESCHERICHIA COLI* ENDOTOXIN IN DBTC- AND DOTC-TREATED RATS[a]

Dietary concentration (ppm)	Number of animals	$\log_2$ Hemagglutination titer in serum	
		Day 7	Day 10
DOTC			
0	5	4.83 ± 1.72	3.50 ± 1.29
50	5	5.11 ± 1.37	3.40 ± 1.34
150	3	4.67 ± 1.08	3.50 ± 0.72
DBTC			
0	5	5.72 ± 0.83	2.84 ± 1.24
50	5	5.84 ± 1.07	3.17 ± 0.98
150	5	4.68 ± 1.07	2.83 ± 1.17

[a] Mean values ± SD. Rats were immunized i.v. with 100 μg of LPS *E. coli* 0 127:B8. Titers were measured 7 and 10 days after immunization according to the method of Andersson and Blomgren.[39]

Table 6
THE EFFECT OF DBTC OR DOTC ON VARIOUS IMMUNE FUNCTIONS OF RATS

	Effect[a]	Ref.
Humoral Immunity		
In vivo	+	24
Thymus-dependent antibody synthesis to sheep red blood cells (SRBC)		
Thymus-independent antibody synthesis to E. coli lipopolysaccharide (LPS)	−	24
In vitro	+	24
Plaque formation against SRBC		
Transformation of lymphocytes by LPS	−	25
Cell Mediated Immunity	+	24
In vivo		
Delayed type hypersensitivity to tuberculin		
Allograft rejection	+	24
Graft vs. host reaction	+	25
Resistance to Listeria monocytogenes infection	+	
In vitro	+	25
Lymphocyte transformation by phytohemagglutinin (PHA) and concanavalin A (Con A)		
Phagocytosis by macrophages of carbon particles	−	24
Sensitivity to LPS	+	

[a] +—Denotes a suppressive effect on immune parameters or an increase of susceptibility to infection or E. coli LPS.

[a] −—No effect.

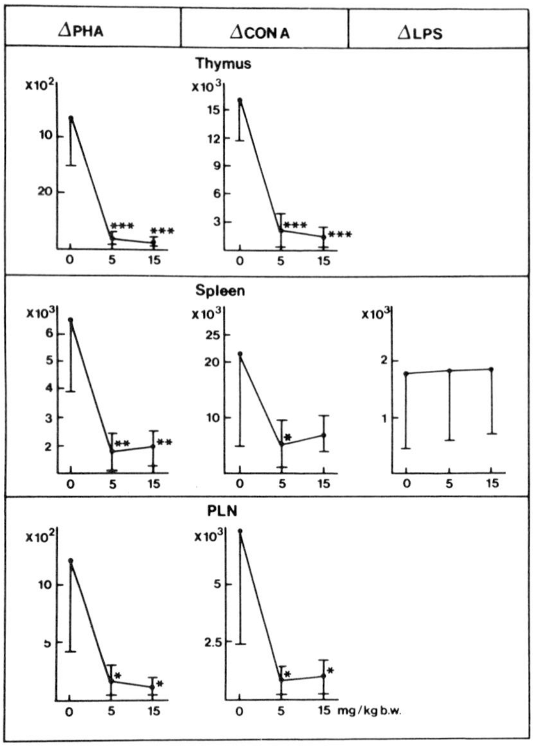

FIGURE 9. Mitogenic response of thymus and spleen cells from littermate rats treated by gavage with 0, 5, or 15 mg DOTC/kg body weight respectively three times a week during four weeks after birth. Results are expressed as the difference of ^{3}H-TdR incorporation between stimulated and unstimulated cultures in cpm per 3 million cells. (Means ± SD, 4—6 animals).

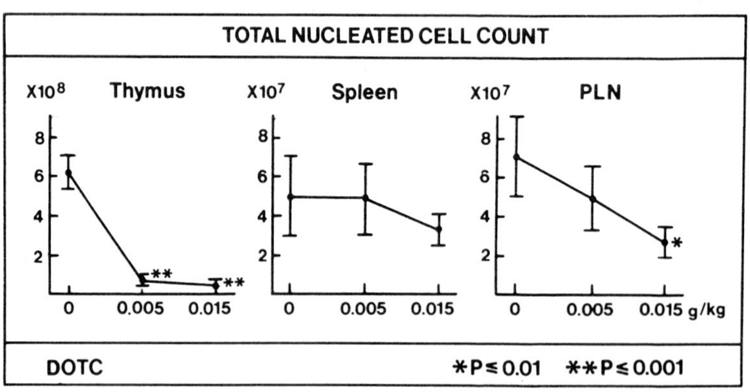

FIGURE 10. Total nucleated cell counts of thymus, spleen, and peripheral lymphnodes from littermate rats treated by gavage with 0, 5, or 15 mg DOTC/kg body weight three times a week during four weeks after birth.

Table 7
MITOGENIC RESPONSE OF THYMUS, SPLEEN, AND PERIPHERAL LYMPHNODE CELLS OF DOTC-TREATED RATS[a]

Dose of DOTC mg/kg	△ PHA[b]	△ Con A[b]	△ LPS[b]
		Thymus	
0	462,000 ± 161,000	3,178,000 ± 885,600	n.d.[c]
5	3,160 ± 1,580[d]	34,800 ± 30,300	n.d.
15	400 ± 210[d]	4,260 ± 3,600	n.d.
		Spleen	
0	179,600 ± 87,800	754,000 ± 554,400	58,740 ± 45,140
5	25,000 ± 21,700[d]	179,400 ± 157,000[e]	58,450 ± 43,250
15	18,700 ± 13,200[d]	141,000 ± 68,800[e]	38,300 ± 26,100
		PLN	
0	27,130 ± 18,480	165,800 ± 110,900	n.d.
5	2,740 ± 1,920[d]	12,900 ± 12,400[d]	n.d.
15	1,180 ± 700[d]	7,780 ± 6,740[d]	n.d.

[a] Littermate rats were dosed with 0 , 5, or 15 mg DOTC/kg bodyweight by gavage three times a week from day 2 after birth until day 27.

[b] Results are expressed as the difference of ^{3}H-thymidine incorporation between stimulated and unstimulated cultures in cpm/organ. Mean values ± SD of 4—6 animals. Twenty hours before the end of the 3-day culture period 0.25 μCi ^{3}H-thymidine (SA 0.5 mCi/mMol) was added to each culture.

[c] Not determined = n.d.

[d] $p < 0.001$.

[e] $p < 0.05$.

V. CONCLUSIONS

From the experiments described in this review it is concluded that some dialkyltin compounds, especially DBTC and DOTC, exert a selective cytotoxic action on T-lymphocytes. As a consequence of this unique phenomenon, atrophy of the lymphoid system occurs and the T-cell-dependent immunity is depressed. Immune suppression is most pronounced in animals exposed to the organotins during the developmental phase of the immune system.

For some organotin compounds, especially DBTC and DOTC, the effects on the immune system are the most sensitive parameters of toxicity. Therefore, a reevaluation of the toxicity of organotin compounds seems to be mandatory, since toxicological studies were made at a time when the immunosuppressive properties were not known.

Since DBTC and DOTC induce immune suppression selectively in those test systems in which T-lymphocytes are predominantly involved, these compounds represent a potential tool for controlling various pathological events in which undesired T-lymphocyte functions are involved.

In contrast to many other cytotoxic drugs, DBTC and DOTC selectively destroy lymphocytes without exerting myelotoxicity or a generalized cytotoxicity and, therefore, may be interesting tools as anti-T-cell tumor compounds.

REFERENCES

1. **Hedges, E. S.,** *Tin in Social and Economic History,* Edward Arnold Ltd., London, 1964.
2. **Löwig, C., Ueber Zinnäthyle, neu aus Zinn und Aethyl bestehende organische Radicale,** *J. Prakt Chem.,* 57, 385, 1852.
3. **Frankland, E.,** Ueber eine neue Reihe organischer Körper, welche Metalle enthalten. *J. Prakt. Chem.,* 58, 421, 61, 208, 1853.
4. **McCabe, W. L. and Meade, B.,** U.S. Patent 1,837,761,1932.
5. **Ingve, V.** U.S. Patent 2,219,463,1940.
6. **Ross, A.,** Industrial application of organotin compounds, *Ann. N.Y. Acad. Sci.,* 125, 107, 1965.
7. **Luyten, J. G. A.,** Applications and biological effects of organotin compounds, in *Organotin Compounds,* Vol. 3, Sawyer, A. K., Ed., Marcel Dekker, New York, 1972, 931.
8. **Van der Kerk, G. J. M.,** Derzeitiger Stand der Anwendungen von Organozinnverbindungen, *Chem. Ztg.,* 99, 26, 1975.
9. **Van der Kerk, G. J. M.,** The organic chemistry of tin, *Chem. Tech.* 8, 356, 1978.
10. **Piver, W. T.,** Organotin compounds: industrial application and biological investigation, *Environ. Health. Perspect.,* 4, 61, 1973.
11. **Van der Kerk, G. J. M.,** Present trends and perspectives in organotin chemistry, *Chem. Ind., London,* 644, 1970.
12. **Barnes, J. M. and Stoner, H. B.,** The toxicology of tin compounds, *Pharmac. Rev.,* 11, 211, 1959.
13. **Alajonanine, T., Derobert, L., and Thieffry, S.,** Etude clinique d'ensemble de 210 cas d'intoxication par les sels organique d'ètain, *Rev. Neurol.,* 98, 85, 1958.
14. **Gruner, J. E.,** Lésions du névraxe secundaire a l'ingestion déthyl-eýtain (Stalinon), *Rev. Neurol.,* 98, 109, 1958.
15. **Magee, P. N., Stoner, H. B., and Barnes, J. M.,** The experimental production of oedema in the central nervous system of the rat by triethyltin compounds, *J. Pathol. Bacteriol.,* 73, 107, 1957.
16. **Klimmer, O. R.,** Die Anwendung von Organozinn-Verbindungen in experimentell-toxicologischer Sicht., *Arzneim. Forsch.,* 19, 934, 1969.
17. **Barnes, J. M. and Stoner, H. B.,** Toxic properties of some dialkyl and trialkyltin salts, *Br. J. Ind. Med.,* 15, 15, 1958.
18. **Cremer, J. E.,** The biochemistry of organotin compounds. The conversion of tetraethyltin into triethyltin in mammals, *Biochem. J.,* 68, 685, 1958.
19. **Stoner, H. B., Barnes, J. M., and Duff, J. I.,** Studies on the toxicity of alkyltin compounds, *Br. J. Pharmacol.,* 10, 16, 1955.
20. **Barnes, J. M. and Magee, P. N.,** The biliary and hepatic lesions produced experimentally by dibutyltin salts, *J. Pathol. Bacteriol.,* 75, 267, 1958.
21. **Klimmer, O. R. and Nebel, I. U.,** Nebel, I. U., Experimentelle Untersuchungen zur Frage der Toxizität einiger Stabilisatoren in Kunststoffen aus Polyvinylchlorid, *Arzneim. Forsch.,* 10, 44, 1960.
22. **Seinen, W. and Willems, M. I.,** Toxicity of organotin compounds. I. Atrophy of thymus and thymus-dependent lymphoid tissue in rats fed di-n-octyltindichloride, *Toxicol. Appl. Pharmacol.,* 35, 63, 1976.
23. **Seinen, W., Vos, J. G., Van Spanje, I., Snoek, M., Brands, R., and Hooykaas, H.,** Toxicity of organotin compounds. II. Comparative in vivo and in vitro studies with various organotin and organolead compounds in different animal species with special emphasis on lymphocyte cytotoxicity, *Toxicol. Appl. Pharmacol.,* 42, 197, 1977.
24. **Seinen, W., Vos, J. G., Van Krieken, R., Penninks, A. H., Brands, R., and Hooykaas, H.,** Toxicity of organotin compounds. III. Suppression of thymus-dependent immunity in rats by di-n-butyltindichloride and di-n-octyltindichloride, *Toxicol. Appl. Pharmacol.,* 42, 213, 1977.
25. **Seinen, W., Vos, J. G., Brands, R., and Hooykaas, H.,** Lymphocytotoxicity and immunosuppression by organotin compounds, Suppression of GVH reactivity, blast transformation and E-rosette formation by di-n-butyltindichloride and di-n-octyltindichloride. *Immuno. Pharmacol.,* 1, 343, 1979.
26. **Seinen, W. and Penninks, A. H.,** Immune suppression as a consequence of a selective cytotoxic activity of certain organometallic compounds on thymus dependent lymphocytes, *Ann. N.Y. Acad. Sci.,* in press, 1979.
27. **Seinen, W.,** Immunotoxicity of Alkyltin Compounds, Ph.D. thesis, University of Utrecht, Utrecht, The Netherlands, 1978.
28. Food and Drug Administration. Appraisal of the safety of chemicals in food, drugs and cosmetics. The Association of Food and Drug Officials of the United States. Austin, 1, Texas, 1959.
29. FAO, Procedures for the testing of intentional food additives to establish their safety for use, *WHO Tech. Rep. Ser.,* no. 144, 1958.
30. FAO/WHO. Procedures for investigating intentional and unintentional food additives, *WHO Tech. Rep. Ser.* no. 348, 1967.

31. **Vos, J. G.,** Immune suppression as related to toxicology, *CRC Crit. Rev. Toxicol.*, 5, 67, 1977.
32. **Voedingsraad,** Algemene richtlijnen voor toevoegingen, Guidelines, Ministry of Health, The Hague, Netherlands, 1973.
33. **Till, J. E. and McCullouch, E. A.,** A direct measurement of the radiation sensitivity of normal mouse bone marrow cells, *Radiat. Res.*, 14, 213, 1961.
34. **Tripathy, S. P. and Mackaness, G. B.,** The effect of cytotoxic agents on the passive transfer of cell mediated immunity, *J. Exp. Med.*, 130, 17, 1969.
35. **Miller, J. F. A. P.,** Effect of neonatal thymectomy on the immunological responsiveness of the mouse, *Proc. Roy. Soc. London Ser. B*, 156, 415, 1961.
36. **Pinto-Machado, J.,** Influence of prenatal administration of busulfan on the postnatal development of mice. Production of a syndrome including hypoplasia of the thymus, *Teratology*, 3, 363, 1970.
37. **Vos, J. G. and Moore, J. A.,** Suppression of cellular immunity in rats and mice by maternal treatment with 2,3,7,8-tetrachlorodibenzo-p-dioxin, *Int. Arch. Allergy. Appl. Immunol.*, 47, 777, 1974.
38. **Ford, W. L., Burr, W., and Simonson, M.,** A lymph node weight assay for the graft-versus-host activity of rat lymphoid cells, *Transplantation*, 10, 258, 1970.
39. **Andersson, B. and Blomgren, H.,** Evidence for thymus-independent humoral antibody production in mice against polyvinyl-pyrrolidone and *E. coli* lipopoly saccharide, *Cell, Immunol.*, 2, 411, 1971.

Chapter 11

ALLERGENS: WITH A SPECIAL REFERENCE TO COMPOSITAE AND FOODS

B. Singh

TABLE OF CONTENTS

I. INTRODUCTION

Allergy is a body reaction that occurs in persons who are sensitive to certain substances. A substance that is harmless to a nonallergic person may cause mild to extremely severe symptoms in an allergic person. A substance that causes an allergy is called an *allergen*. Many allergens are common foods (chocolate, cow's milk, eggs, wheat, shellfish, etc.) or commonly present substances of the environment (house dust, mold spores, pollen, and the dandruff or hair of household pets). The intensity of the reaction depends on the degree of hypersensitivity of the person rather than on the quantity of the allergen.

Allergy is a common affliction. It has been estimated that about 20% of American school children suffer some kind of allergy.[1] Others estimate that 20 million Americans suffer from common allergies; 13 million suffer from hay fever and/or asthma and these people collectively spend some 37 million days a year in bed with their ailments.[2]

II. SYMPTOMS (GENERAL)

Allergic reactions are spontaneous and peculiar to certain persons. The reactions, though triggered by an allergen, are brought about by a certain type of antibody, the *reagin*. There is considerable evidence for a hereditary factor in human allergy, although very little is known about specific genetic factors that are involved. The symptoms are numerous and varied. Almost any tissue of the body may be involved in allergic response (Table 1). The most commonly affected organs are the skin and the respiratory tract which may account for 90% of the disorders of allergy. The gastrointestinal tract is less frequently involved. Food allergy affecting the central nervous system may produce such symptoms as "migraine" and even convulsive seizures. Sometimes allergy to foods may be manifested in the genitourinary tract, in the cardiovascular system, and in the special sense organs.

Allergens find four ways to their sensitive targets: (1) they are inhaled, (2) they are eaten, drunk, or taken as medicine, (3) they are touched or worn, and (4) they are injected into the skin, as by a doctor or the sting of an insect. In general, simple contact with the offending allergen results in skin eruption while inhalation will cause nasal and bronchial symptoms. Ingestion or injection of markedly allergenic foods in highly susceptible individuals sometimes causes minimal local organ or tissue reaction and yet results in profound systemic effect with all the symptoms of shock.

The symptoms vary in speed of onset, in severity, and in duration. They may occur within several minutes and may be violent. In these cases if the cause is not recognized and treated promptly the result may be fatal. Symptoms occurring hours after exposure to the allergen are generally milder and more readily controlled.

III. SENSITIZING AGENTS

Almost any chemical (including food, drug, plant, or animal products) has the capacity to produce an allergic reaction. Some are frequent causes of symptoms while a few, although commonly consumed, touched or inhaled, are rarely implicated. Among the plant foodstuffs as allergens are grains, legumes, and nuts; within animal products, are included eggs, milk, and meat. In the environment, many manmade pollutants and natural products (pollen, spores, molds, hairs, plant parts) may induce allergenic reaction. Hay fever, the most commonly occurring allergy, is caused by airborne pollens and molds. Pollen is produced by different plants in different seasons. In the spring the pollen that causes hay fever is produced by trees such as the elm, birch, maple, ash, oak, poplar, walnut, sycamore, and cypress. In midsummer the hayfever is caused by the pollen from

Table 1
COMMON CLINICAL DISORDERS DUE TO ALLERGY

Human body organs	Type of reaction
Skin	Itchy rash, blisters, sealing, hives, or swelling
Eyes	Unexplained itching, weeping, redness, swelling of eyelids
Digestive tracts	Upset stomach, diarrhea, weight loss, failure to absorb essential nutrients
Respiratory tract	Chronic sinus trouble, sneezing, plugged up ears, irritated throats, hoarseness, stuffed nose, chest congestion, cough and troubled breathing, wheeze of asthma that may lead to more severe conditions

grasses, while in autumn pollen comes from members of the family Compositae. In its season in the Central States and the East alone, ragweed produces about a quarter million tons of pollen.

IV. COMPOSITAE AND CONTACT DERMATITIS

Numerous species of plants produce contact dermatitis. As early as 1894, Mac Dougal[3] published a case of dermatitis due to the showy lady's slipper (*Cypripedium regina, C. spectabile*) and the moccassin flower (*C. calceolus* var. *pubescence*). He also pointed out then a number of native plants which had been definitely ascertained to be more or less poisonous by means of direct contact. Later, Hannah[4] described contact dermatitis due to ragweed. These and many other early observations have been much extended and clarified by (1) immunologic concepts of Bloch and Jadassohn; (2) the chemical and immunobiologic studies of Brown et al.[5] Sulzberger and Wise[73], Brunsting and Anderson[88]; and (3) the clinical studies of Shelmire.[6] Plants and their pollens may be separated into two fractions of clinical importance: (1) the water-soluble protein fraction relating to atopic manifestation such as hay fever, asthma, etc. and (2) the organic solvent fraction (oleoresins) relating to contact dermatitis.

Even though, the chemistry of some plant materials has been studied in considerable detail, immunobiological studies are rather sparse and inconclusive. Brown et al.[5] demonstrated the gross chemical and immunobiological differentiation between the water-soluble protein fraction capable of producing hay fever or asthma and the oleoresin, nonvolatile organic extract fraction capable of producing dermatitis of the contact allergic type. Based on positive patch tests on patients using twenty-four commercial oleoresin weed extracts in acetone, Mackoff and Dahl[7] presented a botanical analysis to establish possible interrelationships and trends. The results indicated that the family Compositae is an outstanding eteological agent in the production of weed contact eczemas. Further analysis revealed that certain tribes within the family Compositae, e.g., sunflower (Helianthiae), dog fennel (Anthemidae) and sneezeweed (Helenieae) are important sources of the sensitizing components (Figure 1). In a given tribe again sensitizing potencies may vary (Figure 2). It has also been concluded that short ragweed contains antigenic substance that shares major antigenic components with false ragweed, burweed, marsh elder, and cocklebur. The tribes Anthemida and Helianthiae provide the majority of cases of oleoresin eczemas (Figure 3 and 4). It has been noted that a patient who is sensitive to the garden *Chrysanthemum* (tribe - Anthemidae) will often react to other

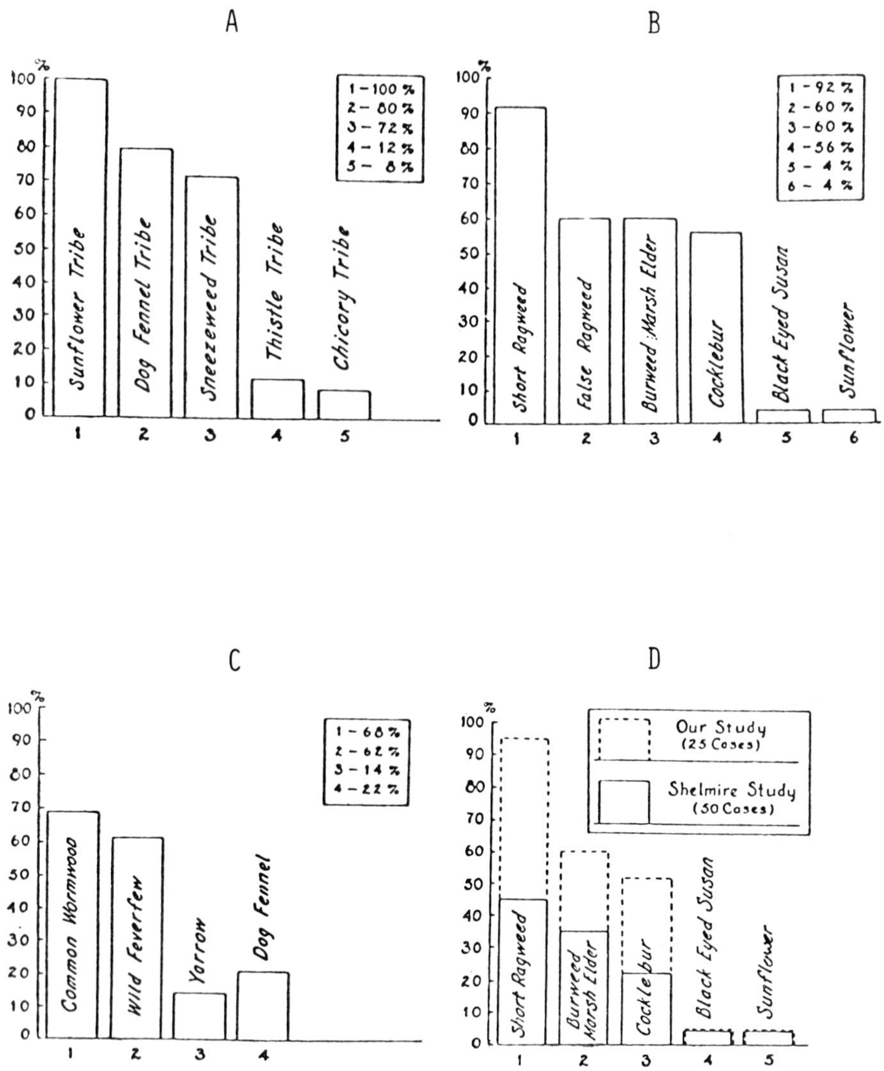

FIGURE 1. Reactions of the family Compositae. (A) Reactions within the family Compositae (%); (B) Reactions within the sunflower tribe (Heliantheae) (%); (C) Reactions within the dog fennel tribe (Anthemidae) (%); (D) Comparative studies: sunflower tribe (Heliantheae) (%). (From Mackoff, S. and Dahl, A. O., Minn. Med., 34, 1169, 1951. With permission.)

genera in the same tribe and to genera in the related tribe (Helianthiae) but rarely to species in other tribes of the Compositae family.[8]

Not all sensitivities to plant materials are immunologically produced. For example, studies indicated that *Arcticum, Matricaria* and *Helium* species have primary irritant properties.[9,10,11] *Archillea* and *Anthemis* species have been reported to cause phytophotodermatitis;[12] however, it is possible that the former is a sensitizer and that the latter is a primary[13,14] irritant, both producing pseudophytophotodermatitis. Mitchell [15] has listed more than 80 species of the compositae family with ability to cause contact dermatitis (Table 2). The commonest sensitizing plants are found in the genera *Ambrosia* and *Chrysanthemum.* In the case of *Ambrosia,* (ragweed species) contact with the plant itself is the most important source of contact sensitivity since droplets of essential oil are present on the surface of the leaves.[8,16] In addition, airborne pollen either contains the

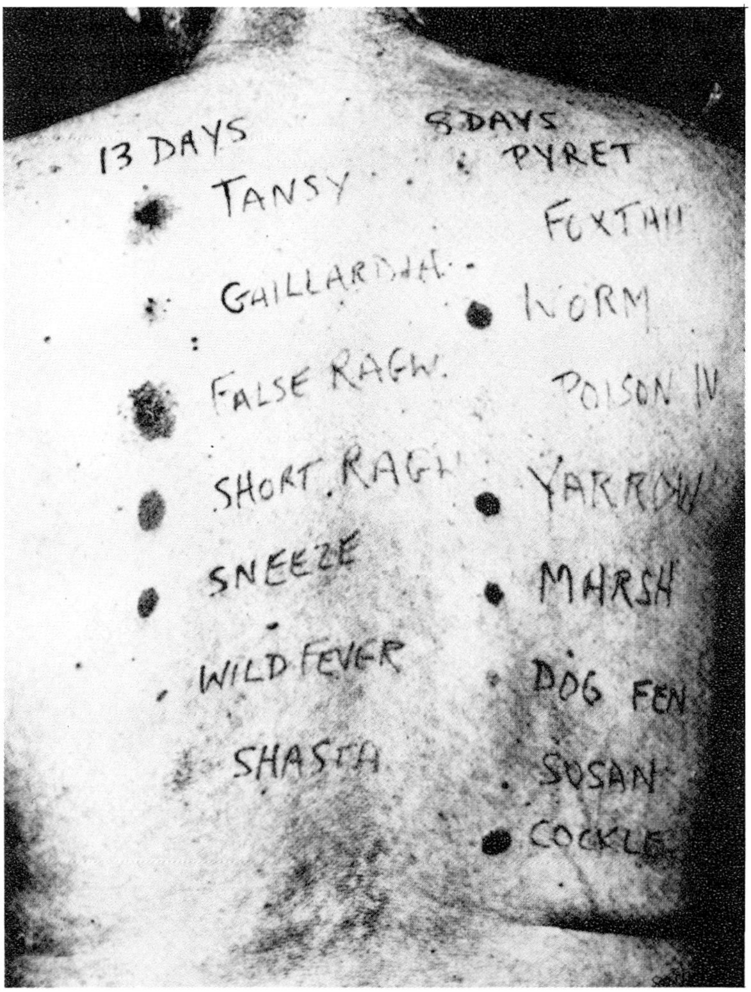

FIGURE 2. Patch test reaction to various members of the family Compositae: 13 days after removal of patches: tansy, gaillardia, shasta daisy 1/10 v/v; false ragweed, short ragweed, sneezeweed, milk feverfew 1/20 v/v, in acetone; 8 days after removal of patches: pyrethrum 10% in petrolatum; foxtail grass, wormwood, yarrow, marshelder, dog fennel, black-eyed Susan, cocklebur 1/10 v/v in acetone; poison ivy 1/50 v/v in acetone. Readings made at 48 hours viz 24 hours after removal of the pathces. (From Mitchell, J. C., Fritig, B., Singh, B., and Towers, G. H. N., *J. Inv. Derm.*, 54, 233, 1970. With permission.)

oil or is contaminated with it. Ragweed oil dermatitis occurs most commonly in farmers between the ages of 40 and 65 years.[17] Seven cases of so-called "milker's eczema" were found to be due to weed oleoresins with which the cow hair was contaminated and not to the cow hair itself.[16]

Epstein[17] has characterized ragweed dermatitis as

1. It is usually an indurated dermatitis with marked chronicity, although active exacerbations are frequent.
2. The clinical picture of chronic cases resembles atopic dermatitis.
3. It often occurs in atopic individuals.

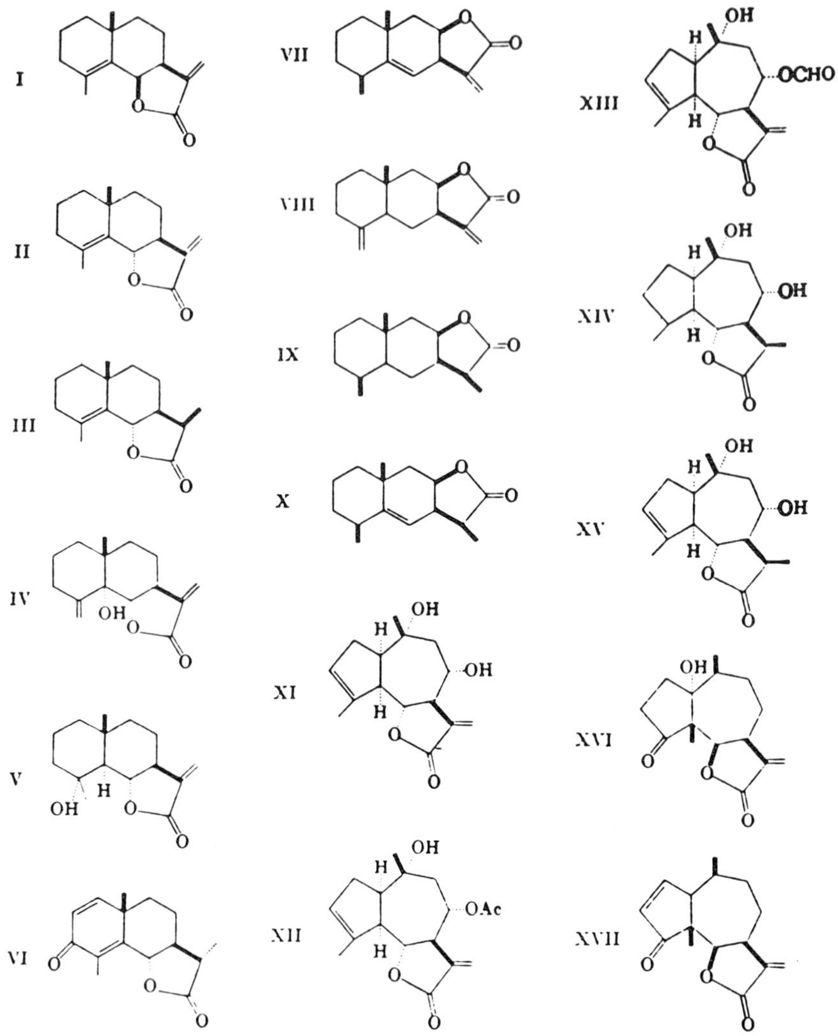

FIGURE 3. Molecular structure of compounds named in Table 3. (From Mitchell, J. C., Fritig, B., Singh, B., and Towers, G. H. N., *J. Inv. Derm.*, 54, 233, 1970. With permission.)

4. Patients react often also to other weeds, especially marsh elder.
5. Dermal contact sensitivity often can be demonstrated.
6. The dermatitis is usually seasonal but may become perennial.

Epstein[17] noted all degrees of patch test reactions to ragweed oleoresin from acute weeping dermatitis to discrete isolated papules. Fromer and Jenkins[18] in a study of 50 cases of ragweed oil dermatitis, observed edematous and erythematous patch test reactions; occasionally vesicles and bullae appeared. Rarely tests were negative at 48 hours but became positive at 5 to 7 days. Fromer and Burrage[19] observed that positive patch test reactions persisted for up to 7 weeks. Shelmire[16] observed that application of the plant leaf for 1 hour was sufficient to produce a positive reaction in a sensitized patient. In a report on ragweed dermatitis by Brunsting and Williams,[20] 40 of 44 patients were males. This may perhaps be due to the frequency of exposure.

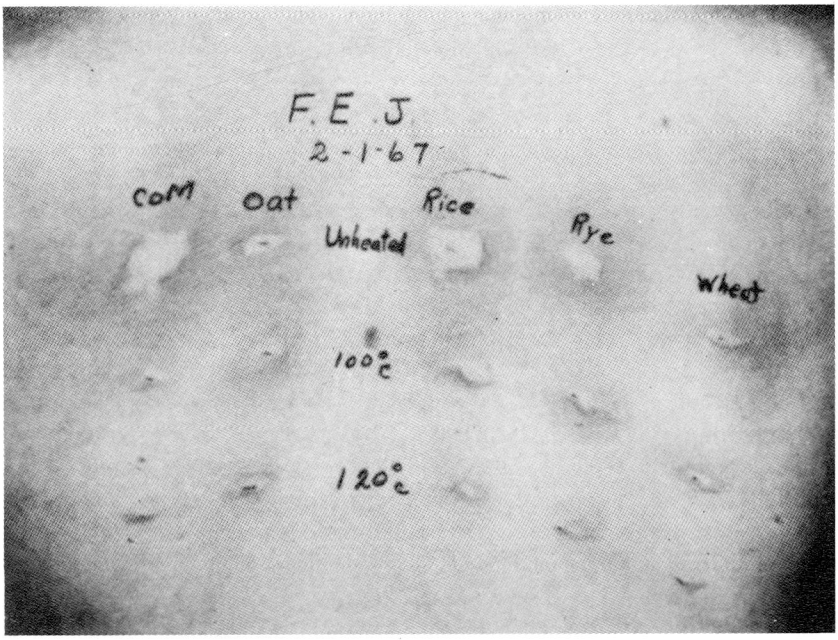

FIGURE 4. Reactions to various legumes (left back) and grains (right back) showing effect of heat on these extracts which in unheated state gave strong skin test reactions. (From Pearlman, F., *Toxic Constituents of Plants,* Liener, I. E., Ed., Academic Press, New York, 1969. With permission.)

Table 2
COMPOSITAE SPECIES LISTED BY BOTANICAL NAME AND COMMON NAME; REFERENCES IN LITERATURE TO CONTACT DERMATITIS FROM EXPOSURE TO THESE PLANTS[a]

	Sub-family: Asteroideae (Tubuliflorae)	
Genus and Species	**Common Name**	**Ref.**
	Tribe 1: Heliantheae	
Ambrosia spp.	Ragweed spp.	17, 5, 72
A. artemesifolia	Short ragweed, low ragweed	20, 73
A. bidentata	Southern ragweed, Lance-leaved ragweed	16, 6
A. eliator	Common ragweed, short ragweed	6, 16
A. psilostachya	Western ragweed	6, 16
A. trifida	Giant ragweed, tall ragweed	16
Cosmos bipinnatus		74
Cyclachaena xanthifolia	Burweed marshelder, giant poverty weed, horseweed, prairie ragweed	20
Encelia californica		75
Franseria acanthicarpa	False ragweed, poverty weed, bur	7, 74
Gaillardia spp.	Gaillardia	31, 16
G. picta		76
G. pulchella	Fire weed	16
Galinsoja parviflora		77
Helenium autumnale	Sneezeweed, false sunflower	7
H. microcephalum	Sneezeweed, false sunflower	16
H. tenuifolium	Bitterweed	16

Table 2 (continued)
COMPOSITAE SPECIES LISTED BY BOTANICAL NAME AND COMMON NAME; REFERENCES IN LITERATURE TO CONTACT DERMATITIS FROM EXPOSURE TO THESE PLANTS[a]

Genus and Species	Sub-family: Asteroideae (Tubuliflorae)	
	Common Name	**Ref.**
	Tribe 1: Heliantheae	
Helianthus annuus	Sunflower	76
Iva augustifolia	Narrow leaf marshelder	6, 16
I. axillaris	Poverty weed, small-flowered marshelder	6, 16
I. ciliata	Rough marshelder	80
I. xanthifolia	Burweed Marshelder	16
Oxytenia acerosa	Copper weed	81
Parthenium argentatum	Guayule, Mexican rubber plant	82
Parthenium hysterophorus	Feverfew	16
Rudbeckia hirta	Black-eyed Susan	7
Rudbeckia serotina		7
Xanthium canadense or *pennsylvanicum*	Cocklebur, clotbur	7, 16, 20
X. spinosum		6
X. strumarium		6
	Tribe 2: Astereae	
Aster exilis	Aster, Michaelmas daisy	16
A. multiflorus	Aster, Michaelmas daisy	16, 75
Cassinia aculeata	Dogweed, Australian dogweed	83
Erigeron philadelphicus	Fleabane	16
Solidago virga aurea	Golden rod (carries extraneous pollen)	79
	Tribe 3: Anthemidae	
Achillea lanulosa	Yarrow	7
A. millefolium	Milfoil, yarrow, nose bleed	7, 82
Anthemis cotula	Stinking mayweed, dog fennel	7, 84
A. Arvensis	Corn chamomile	38, 79
A. nobilis	Chamomile (Camomile)	16
Artemesia cina, maritima	(Santonin)	27
A. ludoviciana	Western mugwort, prairie sage	7
A. vulgaris	Common mugwort	7
Chrysanthemum spp.		74
C. cinerariaefolium	Dalmatian chrysanthemum, Japanese daisy, Persian insect powder	79
C. coccineum	Pyrethrum roseum, painted daisy, Persian insect powder	20
C. indicum		
	Tribe 3: Anthemidae	
C. leucanthemum	Marguerite, whiteweed, ox-eye daisy, King Edward daisy	7
C. marshallicarneum		79
C. maximum	Shasta daisy	16
C. x-morifolium	Chrysanthemum of florists	10, 23
C. parthenium	Feverfew	6, 16
C. roseum	Pyrethrum	79
Matracaria spp.	Chamomile	77
Tanacetum vulgare	Tansy	19, 23

Table 2 (continued)
COMPOSITAE SPECIES LISTED BY BOTANICAL NAME AND COMMON NAME; REFERENCES IN LITERATURE TO CONTACT DERMATITIS FROM EXPOSURE TO THESE PLANTS[a]

Genus and Species	Common Name	Ref.
	Sub-family: Asteroideae (Tubuliflorae)	
	Tribe 5: Inuleae	
Inula graveolens	Stinkwort	83
	Tribe 6: Senecioneae	
Arnica montana	Mountain tobacco, leopard's bane	39, 79, 82, 90, 105
Cineraria martima	Seaside ragwort	86
Doronicum spp.	Thistle family	86
D. Pardalianches	Roman leopard's bane	86
Senecio cineraria	Dusty miller	86
	Tribe 7: Calenduleae	
Calendula tagetes	Marigold (Legion of Honour)	86
	Tribe 8: Eupatorieae	
Eupatorium serotinum	Boneset	16
	Tribe 9: Vernonieae	
Veronia baldwinii		
	Tribe 10: Cynareae	
Arctium lappa	Great burdock, burdock	84, 86
Cryptostemma calendulaceum	Cape-weed (native of South Africa, adventive to Australia)	83
Cyanara scolymus	Globe artichoke	86
	Sub-family: Lactucoideae (Liguliflorae)	
	Tribe 12: Lactuceae (Cichorieae)	
Lactuca sativa	Lettuce	86
Taraxacum officinale	Dandelion[b]	87

[a] Adopted from Mitchell[15]
[b] Reported to cross-react with *Apium graveolens*, celery and *Anthemis nobilis*.

In certain cases of ragweed dermatitis a combination of plain contact allergy and photo contact allergy may be evident.[14,17,19] There is an apparent association of ragweed oil dermatitis and atopic dermatitis. For example, Jillson et al.[21] found that six patients with ragweed oil dermatitis were atopic subjects and thus concluded that atopy predisposed to this type of allergic contact dermatitis. Fromer and Burrage[19] noted that 2 out of 25 patients with ragweed oil dermatitis were atopic subjects. He observed that ragweed oil dermatitis affects the extensor aspects of the upper limbs and the distribution pattern is quite unlike that of atopic dermatitis. It is quite possible that atopic individuals are in double jeopardy. They have a chance of developing contact dermatitis and a chance of also developing atopic dermatitis or both concurrently for an entirely nonimmunologic reason. Individuals with atopic dermatitis are more likely to become sensitized to simple chemicals because their skin is inflamed and is the more likely to be the site of induction of a sensitization process.

Ragweed oil dermatitis is the most prevalent form of pollen dermatitis in the U.S. and Canada. However, other weeds among the compositae are reported to be associated with pollen contact sensitization (*Xanthium, Erigeron, Iva* sps.). Ragweed is not found in Australia but cape weed (*Cryptestemma*), an adventive in Australia from South Africa, is a common cause of hay fever. Cape weed may cause contact dermatitis and photosensitivity.[22] Ragweed species are only adventives in Britain. Rook[23] observed positive patch test reactions to *Xanthimum* and to *Chrysanthemum.* Dermatitis may occur in florists, gardeners, and others who handle the plant.[23] Pyrethrum has been used as an insecticide and dermatitis is common in East Africa among workers employed in its manufacture.

Hjorth and Fregret[25] suggested that probably most plant allergens comprise several substances which are cross-sensitive to their chemical precursors and degradation products. Cross-reactions between Compositae are the rule. However, contact dermatitis from *Chrysanthemum* may be specific to a single species.[10] Shelmire[16] observed a patient who reacted to *Parthenium* extract in a 1 in 100,000 dilution but showed no patch test reaction to 68 other common weeds. Mitchell[15] reported a case where a white male logger, aged 64 years, had recurrent dermatitis of the exposed skin surfaces for 45 years. For 40 years, the dermatitis occurred only during work in forest areas; in the 5 years after he retired from the forest industry, dermatitis appeared during July to October when he was at home. He became a *Chrysanthemum* fancier after retirement and he was of the opinion that he was allergic to some plant in the woods which he could not identify and to *Chrysanthemum.* This turned out to be right (Figure 5). Positive patch test reactions were observed to some plants of the tribes Heliantheae and Anthemidae. The patient also reacted to *Chrysanthemum* sp., alantolactone derived from *Inula helenium* and to *Frullania nisqualleusis,* one of seven species of liverworts known to occur in forest areas of British Columbia.

In an investigation, on some sensitizing agents for workers in forest industries of British Columbia, Mitchell et al.[26] observed 15 cases of allergic contact dermatitis from Frullania, a genus of liverworts. In five patients so tested, positive patch test reactions have also been obtained from some species of the tribes Heliantheae and Anthemidae of the compositae family. This turned out to be an interesting study in elucidating the role or sesquiterpene lactones in contact dermatitis.[27,28]

V. CHEMICAL BASIS OF CONTACT DERMATITIS TO COMPOSITAE

Sesquiterpene lactones are commonly found in compositae but only occur to a small extent outside this family of flowering plants. The active sesquiterpene lactone present in *Frullania nisquallensis* was an eudesmanolide (Table 3; Fig. 6). In a study, Mitchell et al.[27] tested various sesquiterpene lactones which had been isolated from members of the compositae. The results indicated that the allergenic properties of Compound I are shared by other sesquiterpene lactones because, among the 17 lactones tested, 10 gave positive reactions. The most allergenic lactone was found to be alantolactone (VII), the oldest known sesquiterpene lactone.

Mitchell et al.[27] further noted that the eudesmanolide class of lactones, both of the santonin-type and the alantolactone-type is of particular interest. These lactones pro-

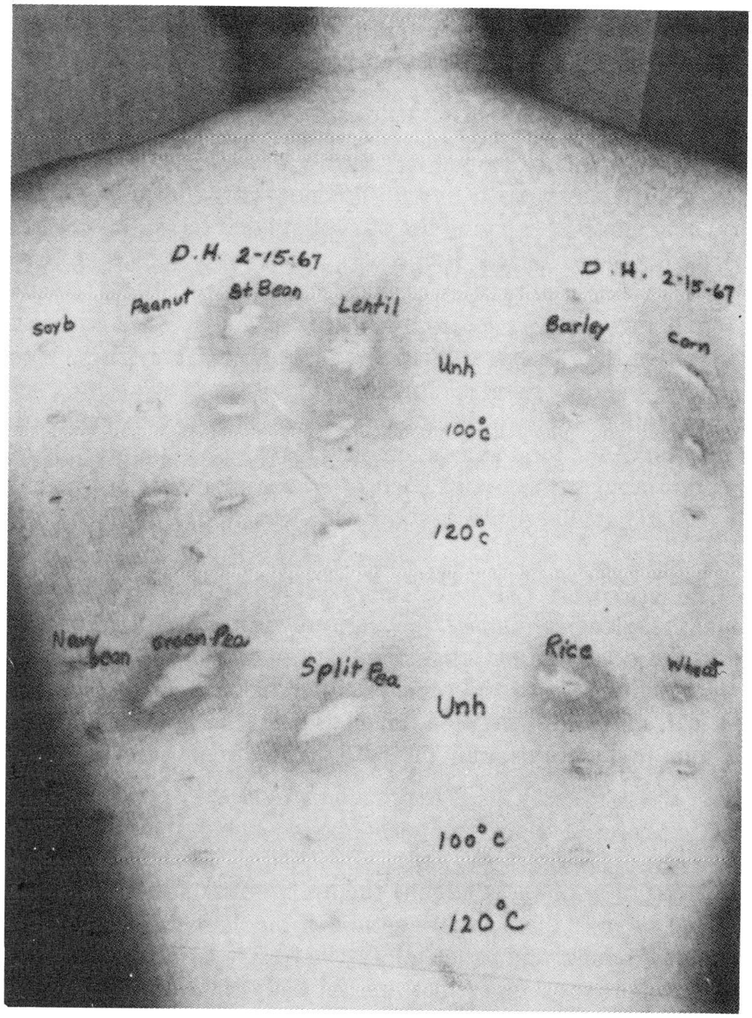

FIGURE 5. Varying degree of skin test reactions to grains with reduction of such reaction after heating to 100°C for 30 min and complete abolition of reactions after heating to 120°C for 20 min. (From Pearlman, F., *Toxic Constituents of Plants*, Liener, I. E., Ed., Academic Press, New York, 1969. With permission.)

duced positive patch test responses. On the contrary, the lactones of the guanolide and pseudoguanolide classes produced positive patch test responses in only a few cases. They are also less active at higher concentrations. It is probable that haptens are bound to one or more proteins and, consequently, there may be some consistent structural requirements for the allergenic activity of these lactones. The active compounds noted above are represented in different classes and it may be observed that a specific skeleton is not a basic requirement for allergenic activity. Within each class, lactones differed only in some simple functional group, such as an additional hydroxyl group, acetylation, or formylation of a hydroxyl group; addition of an exocyclic or endocyclic carbon-carbon double bond, and migration or hydrogenation of one or two double bonds. Only one common structural requirement was found, viz., the presence of a conjugated lactone group. Where the exocyclic carbon-carbon double bond conjugated with the carbonyl is reduced, there is a loss of allergenic activity. In another study, Mitchell and Dupuis[29]

Table 3
PATCH TEST REACTIONS TO CHEMICALS DERIVED FROM *FRULLANIA* AND COMPOSITAE[a]

Class	Number[b]	Name	Vehicle 80% ethyl alcohol conc. (mg/mℓ)	Patch test results Case 1	2	3	4	5
Eudesmanolides (santonin-type)	I	Not yet named	250	2			3	4
	II	Arbusculin-B	200	2			3	3
	III	Dihydroarbusculin-B	400	0			0	0
	IV	Not yet named	400	4			3	4
	V	Arbusculin-A	200	2			3	3
	VI	α-Santonin	1000	0			0	0
Eudesmanolides (alantolactone-type)	VII	Alantolactone	80	3	2	1	4	4
	VIII	Isoalantolactone	200	0		0	0	1
	IX	Tetrahydroalantolactone	400	0			0	0
	X	Dihydroalantolactone	400	0			0	0
Guaianolides	XI	Cumambrin B	400	3			2	0
	XII	Cumambrin A	400	3			1	0
	XIII	Formylcumambrin B	400	4			2	0
	XIV	Tetrahydrocumambrin B	400	0			0	0
	XV	Dihydrocumambrin B	400	0			0	0
Pseudoguaianolides	XVI	Coronopilin	400	2			0	1
	XVII	Ambrosin	400	3			0	0

[a] Delayed. Adapted from Mitchell et al.[27]
[b] Refers to numbering in Figure 3.

tested 52 lactones derived from various species of compositae and suggested that such lactones are responsible for allergic contact dermatitis by ragweed (*Ambrosia*), feverfew (*Parthenium*), sneezeweed (*Helenium*), sagebrush, wormwood, mugwort (*Artmesia*), boneset (*Eupatorium*), povertyweed (*Fransenia*), Marshelder (*Iva*), cocklebur (*Xanthium*), curdock (*Arctium*), chamomile (*Anthemis*), artichoke (*Cynara*), and gaillardia and *Chrysanthemum* species (tansy, pyrethrum).

Allergic contact dermatitis tends to be immunologically specific, that is, the allergic patients react only to a single chemical or to a group of closely related chemicals. Thus, Mitchell[30] found that a human subject who is allergic to usnic acid will react to lichens containing usnic acid but not to lichens which do not contain usnic acid. Further, allergenicity is known to be stereoisomerically specific. In one study, the patients were tested with racemic and with d- and l-usnic acid by standard 24 hour occlusive patch tests. Positive reactions were observed to racemic and to d-usnic acid but not to l-usnic acid. Rostenburg and Good,[31] in a discussion of the pathogenesis of allergic contact dermatitis, concluded that the requisite of a simple chemical capable of acting as a hapten is that it is able to attach to the surface of a protein molecule with a relative ease but not markedly affect the integrity of the protein. In the guinea pig, skin sensitization to simple chemicals, e.g., picryl chloride, is assumed to be due to a conjugation with the free-NH_2 groups of lysine.

VI. FOOD ALLERGENS

Allergic reactions to foods are spontaneously occurring disorders in sensitive individuals. This allergic reaction is an immunologic phenomenon identified as antigen (allergen) - antibody (reagin) reaction. The antigen may be pure protein or a protein

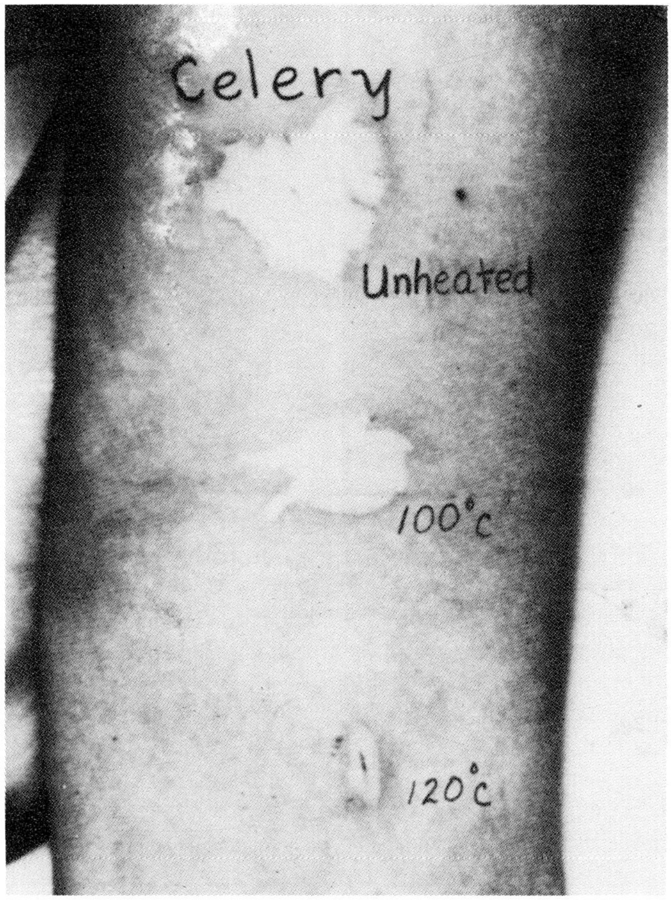

FIGURE 6. Effect of heat on celery extract showing slight reduction of allergenicity after heating to 100°C for 30 min and abolition of skin test reaction after heating to 120°C for 20 min. (From Pearlman, F., *Toxic Constituents of Plants,* Liener, I. E., Ed., Academic Press, New York, 1969. With permission.)

conjugated to a nonantigenic fraction. In sensitive humans, the symptoms are peculiar to the target organ which is involved and, since all body tissues may be affected at one time or another, such symptoms are protean.[32] The target organs most frequently affected are the skin, the respiratory system, and the gastrointestinal tract. Other tissues and organs may be involved.

The foods to which children and adults are most generally sensitive are the common foods such as milk, eggs, wheat, beans, tomatoes, and chocolate. These foods have two things in common.[33] In the first place, they have been introduced into the diet at an early age and are taken in large quantity. Also in the case of milk, eggs, wheat, and beans there is a high concentration of foreign protein present. Proteins were originally thought to be absolutely necessary for antigenic activity, that is, the production of antibodies or sensitization. However, other groups of chemicals are recently found to be strong sensitizers.

When antigenic proteins are broken down by acid or enzymatic hydrolysis as would be present in the digestive tract they become less antigenic and can loose all functional antigenicity when split into very small molecular components. It seems probable, therefore, that most foods are nonantigenic after digestion; but in the individual with a predisposition to acquire sensitivity, the absorption of undigested food through the intestinal mucosa undoubtedly is the seat of sensitization.[33]

Although biochemical studies have been done on many foods, adequate characterization of the allergens has not been adequately investigated. It has been recognized though, that these allergens are large molecular weight substances that are not dialyzable and are most often identified with protein fraction.[34] Further, food proteins of large molecular weight are very antigenic. Pure fatty fractions of food do not cause reactions either clinically or immunologically, and, if any skin test reactions occur in a highly sensitive person, one must suspect some contamination with protein.[35] The important role which polysaccharides may play as antigens was shown first in various types of pneumococci. In many foods, there is probably a protein-carbohydrate complex which is actively allergenic. A purified polysaccharide, levan, a polymer of fructose was injected into humans by Allen and Kabat[36] and an antibody was produced. The anti-levan from one such serum was partially precipitated by rye grass levan. This raises the important question of cross reactivity in foods.

Some low molecular weight compounds have been found to be allergenic. For example, nordihydroguaiaretic acid is an antioxidant used as a food additive in fats. It has been found to produce marked sensitization.[37] It has been suggested that the binding to tissue proteins probably takes place in the catechol residue. Freedman et al.[38] found chlorogenic acid extracted from the green coffee as a sensitizing agent in workers in coffee industry. These workers developed occupational rhinitis and bronchial asthma. It was suggested that chlorogenic acid might be the active allergen in other plant parts responsible for allergic reactions in humans. In fact, chlorogenic acid is present in most fruits.

In many cases, chemical contaminants in foods may be the cause of allergic reaction in certain patients. For example, foods which have been contaminated by petro-, sulfo-, chloro-, and other halogenated compounds are often good sensitizers.[39] Randolph[39] found that the patients who were clinically sensitive to peaches were able to tolerate unsprayed, unsulfured, and wormy peaches. The same was true for the ingestion of dates and figs. When these foods were fumigated with methylbromide, severe reactions occurred in allergic individuals. It is, therefore, important to recognize that the patient, supposedly allergic to a food, may actually be sensitive to the contaminant on the food, such as fungicides, insectides, or herbicides. Milk, in particular, has been contaminated and can cause allergic reactions because, the contaminant, for example, sulfanilamide, penicillin, cottonseed meal, and linseed meal was administered to the cow.

VII. STABILITY OF THE FOOD ALLERGEN

In order to produce allergic reaction, the allergen must show stability through harvesting, storing, processing, and preparation in the kitchen. In addition, it should survive through ingestion, digestion, and final intestinal absorption of a sufficient quantity of allergenic material to reach the shock organ containing a specific reaginic antibody.[40] Some foods lose their allergenicity in the course of harvesting and processing. With these foods only growers and processors are affected. Other foods do not lose their allergenicity through processing, preparation, or ingestion.

The effect of heat on stability of allergens has been studied in a number of foods. Malkin and Markow[41] found no difference in 91% of tests made with raw vs. cooked foods. Pearlman[35] studied the effect of heat with grains, legumes, and a number of other foods and found no consistency in stability of allergens as measured by the skin test (Figure 6,7). Saperstein and Anderson[42] tested a number of liquid and powdered infant milk preparations which were subjected to temperatures of 110°C for 10 min, or 90°C

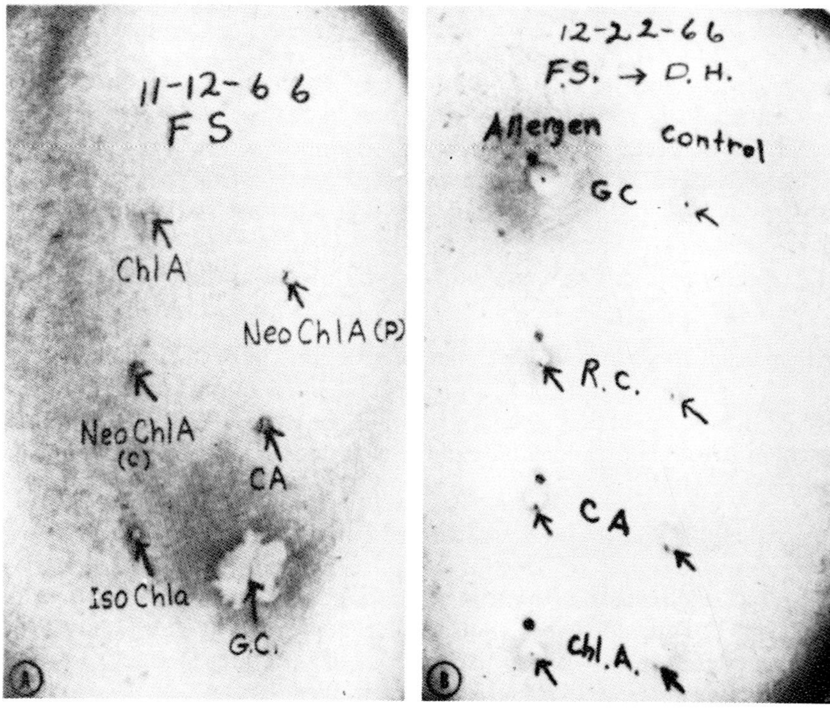

FIGURE 7. Skin test reactions with various fractions of coffee demonstrating that the allergen is in the nondialyzable retentate and is thermolabile. Pure chlorogenic acid failed to give skin reaction. (A) Direct testing with chlorogenic acid from coffee (Ch A), neochlorogenic acid from prunes "Neo Chlo A (P)", neochlorogenic acid from coffee "New Chlo A (C)", caffeic acid (CA), isocholorogenic acid from coffee (Iso Chlo), and green coffee retentate (GC). Only the nondialyzable green coffee reacted. (B) Indirect (passive transfer) testing using serum of patient in A on a non-allergic recipient; green coffee (GC), roasted coffee (RC), caffeic acid (CA), chlorogenic acid (pure) (Chl A). (From Pearlman, F., *Toxic Constituents of Plants,* Liener, I. E., Ed., Academic Press, New York, 1969. With permission.)

for 30 min. By means of the ring precipitaion test and passive cutaneous anaphylaxis in guinea pigs, it was demonstrated that a reduction, but not a complete loss, in antigenicity of the alpha-lactalbumin protein took place but no such alteration in the antigenicity of casein and beta-lactoglobulin portions was observed. The bovine serum albumin and bovine gamma globulin portions, however, were inactivated to a large measure by the heating process. This indicated the complex nature of antigenic components which may be present in a single food. A few foods show invariable thermolability. This is best exemplified with coffee[35] (Figure 7).

Vaughan and Black[43] classified foods botanically for use in allergic diagnosis instead of the culinary classification. Evidence of crossed allergic reactions to foods within a botanical group was found and many foods which would seem similar to the layman appear quite scattered in different generic groups. Baldwin and Benedict[44] have presented experimental evidence of a chemical and immunological crossed relationship and this was confirmed by Withers.[45] Table 4 lists various foods of vegetable origin and their allergenicity to humans.

Table 4
FOOD GROUPS AND THEIR ALLERGENICITY

Food group	Allergenicity	Allergenic principle	Ref.
Cereals	By inhalation, contact, ingestion		
Wheat	Inhalation, contact or ingestion (Baker's Eczema)	Albumin, thermolabile	46
Corn	Ingestion, quite frequent	Uncharacterized protein, fairly thermostable	47
Rice	Ingestion, quite frequent	Protein, thermolabile	35
Oat	Rarely allergenic substitute for wheat and other grains in allergic individuals	—	—
Barley	Allergenic, quite frequent	Protein, thermostable	35
Buckwheat	Contact, ingestion	Protein	48, 49, 50
Vegetables			
Legumes (Peanut, lentin, peas)	Ingestion	Protein, thermolabile and stable	51
Soybeans	Ingestion or contact, frequent	Protein, thermostable	52, 53
Fruits	Ingestions	Protein	54
Banana	Ingestions	Thermolabile	55
Pineapple	Ingestions	Chlorogenic Acid	38
Mango	Ingestions	Chlorogenic Acid	38
Nuts			
Coconut, cashews, etc.	Ingestion, frequent	Protein	35
Seeds	Most highly allergenic food groups		
Cottonseed	Ingestion	Protein	57
Castor bean	Inhalation, ingestion, frequent	Protein	50, 51
Mustard seed	Ingestion	Protein, thermolabile	35
Sesame, poppy, caraway, and anise seeds	Ingestion	Protein, thermolabile	35
Beverages			
Chocolate	Ingestion, contact	Protein, thermolabile	59
Coffee (green)	Inhalation, ingestion	Protein, thermolabile	60
Tea	None	—	—
Carbonated "Soft" beverages	Ingestion, infrequent	Additives used for flavoring or coloring	35
Beer	Ingestion, contact	Malt, hops, yeast, protein	35
Alcoholic distillates	None	—	—
Yeast and Molds	Inhalant allergents	Protein	35
Milk	Ingestion, frequent	Protein, thermostable	61
Meat, Poultry, Fish	Ingestion, frequent	Protein, thermolabile	70

VIII. IMMUNOLOGIC ASPECTS OF ALLERGY

The allergic reaction is brought about by a certain type of antibody, called reagins. It differs from the other humoral antibody which can be developed in the experimental animal and which are associated with anaphylaxis. Pearlman and Layton[63] pointed out two major differences, namely, the thermolability of the reaginic antibodies and their capacity to sensitize passively the skin of nonallergic humans and subhuman primates.

The skin-sensitizing capacity of reagin is used in detecting the allergy. Since the reaginic antibody is found in the serum, and thus in the tissue, its presence can be demonstrated by the introduction of the specific allergen. The presence of reagin can be further demonstrated by transferring serum from the allergic person to the skin of nonallergic humans or subhuman primates.[50,64,65,66] The reagins are probably a heterogeneous group having no single position among the immunoglobulins. The reagin titer is not always correlated with patients sensitivity.

Thermostable (blocking) antibodies are circulating antibodies found in persons who have received a series of injections of a specific antigen. They can be produced in nonallergic as well as in allergic persons receiving such antigen injections. These antibodies are heat stable and can be separated from the skin sensitizing antibodies which are readily destroyed by heating to 60°C for one hour.[35] The molecular size of the thermostable antibodies permits their passage across the placental barrier and their appearance in cord blood. These antibodies do not sensitize skin but rather compete with skin sensitizing antibody itself for the specific antigen.

Cellular antibodies are associated with delayed hypersensitivity leading to contact dermatitis. These antibodies are presumed to be in the cells rather in the serum and are usually identified with the mononuclear leukocytes.

IX. DETECTION OF ALLERGENS

Allergists can use several methods to detect offending substances. An experienced physician may determine the cause by permitting the patient to recount symptoms in relation to food intake. Alternatively, a diet diary is maintained by a careful listing of the ingested food together with a record of symptoms experienced. This is done for days or even weeks.

The elimination diet method is practiced where diets are reduced to a few basic foods and relationship to relief of symptoms is noted.[64] In provocative methods suspected foods are well disguised and are administered in an attempt to reproduce symptoms.[65] However, this may be a hazardous procedure when highly allergenic foods are involved.

A number of objective methods have been used to detect allergy. This includes skin test either by the scratch or intracutaneous method. Pearlman[32] points out that for immunologic diagnosis, food allergens should have the following qualities.. (1) the material should have sufficient concentration to excite the immunological response; (2) it should be free from unknown contaminating allergens; (3) it should be free from nonspecific irritants; (4) it should be in a stable form retaining its antigenicity for a designated period of time; and (5) it should have designated measure of potency. Too often these requirements are not met. Several methods have been proposed for extraction, preservation and administration of allergens to the skin.[66,67]

Several other methods have been proposed for specific diagnosis of offending allergens. For example, (1) Basophil degranulation as proposed by Shelley,[68] (2) release of histamine from leukocytes and from human or lower primate tissue,[69] and (3) the lymphocyte transformation test.[70] Most of the diagnostic methods have little practical value.

X. CONTACT DERMATITIS

In the case of contact dermatitis, portions of suspected material are used for patch testing. Patches are normally removed after 24 hours and reactions are read at 24, 48 hours, 5, and 14 days and scored.[71] Patch testing with chemicals is carried out with solvents (such as 80% ethanol). Isolation of allergens is normally carried out using standard chemical procedures (fractionation, extraction, chromatography, and identification by instrumental methods). For example, for isolation of the causal agent in *Frullania nisquallensis* the plant material was ground up and extracted several times with ethyl ether.[27] Chromatography of the ether extract was carried out with silica-gel as adsorbent. Several runs with various concentrations of ether in petroleum ether as eluant were performed and final purification was achieved by fractional sublimation. Identification was made by further chemical tests, derivatization, and spectroscopy.

REFERENCES

1. **Arbeiter, H. I.,** How prevalent is allergy among United States school children, *Clin. Pediatr.*, 6, 140, 1967.
2. **Clamon, L. N.,** *Allergy: Its Mysterious Causes and Modern Treatment*, Grosset and Dunlap, New York, 1967.
3. **MacDougal, D. T.,** Poisonous influences of various species of Cypripedium, *Minnesota Botan.*, Studies, 32, 450, 1894.
4. **Hannah, L.,** Ragweed dermatitis - a new treatment with preliminary report of a case, *JAMA*, 22, 8535, 1919.
5. **Brown, A., Milford, E. L., and Coca, A. F.,** Studies in contact dermatis. I. The nature and etiology of pollen dermatis, *J. Immunol.*, 20, 301, 1931.
6. **Shelmire, B.,** Contact dermatitis from weeds. Patch testing with their oleoresins, *JAMA*, 113, 1085, 1939.
7. **Mackoff, S. and Dahl, A. O.,** A botanical consideration of the weed oleoresin problem, *Minn. Med.*, 34, 1169, 1951.
8. **Rook, A.,** Plant dermatitis — botanical aspects, *Trans. St. John's Hosp. Derm. Soc.*, 46, 41, 1961.
9. **Templeton, H. J.,** Epidermal and dermal sensitization (coexisting in the same individual), *JAMA*, 127, 908, 1945.
10. **Rook, A.,** Plant dermatitis. The significance of variety specific sensitization, *Brit. J. Derm.*, 73, 283, 1961.
11. **Pascher, F. and Sulzberger, M. B.,** Ragweed dermatitis. Report of two cases, *Arch. Derm. and Syph.*, 28, 223, 1933.
12. **Bellringer, H. E.,** Phyto-photo-dermatitis, *Br. Med. J.*, 1, 984, 1949.
13. **Van Dijk, E. and Berrens, L.,** Plants as an etiological factor in phytophotodermatitis, *Dermatologica*, 129, 321, 1964.
14. **Van Dijk, E.,** Milestones in dermatology. LVIII. Phytophotodermatitis, *Excerpta Med., Sect. 13:* 18, 371, 1964.
15. **Mitchell, J. C.,** Allergic contact dermatitis from compositae, *Trans. St. John's Hospital Dermatological Soc.*, 55, 174, 1969.
16. **Shelmire, B.,** Contact dermatitis from weeds. Patch testing with their oleoresins, *South. Med. J.*, 33, 337, 1940.
17. **Epstein, S.,** Role of dermal sensitivity in ragweed contact dermatitis, *Arch. Derm.*, 82, 48, 1960.
18. **Fromer, J. L. and Jenkins, W. S.,** Ragweed oil dermatitis, *Lahey Clinic Bull.*, 11, 75, 1959.
19. **Fromer, J. L. and Burrage, W. S.,** Ragweed oil dermatitis, *J. Allergy*, 24, 425, 1953.
20. **Brunsting, L. A. and Williams, D. H.,** Ragweed (contact) dermatitis. Observations in 48 cases and report of unsuccessful attempts at desensitization by injection of specific oils, *JAMA*, 106, 1533, 1936.
21. **Jillson, O. F., Curwen, W. L., and Alexander, B. R.,** Problems of contact dermatitis in the atopic individual: with reference to neomycin and ragweed oil sensitivity, *Ann. Allergy*, 17, 215, 1959.
22. **Rook, A.,** Plant dermatitis, *Br. Med. J.*, 2, 1771, 1966.
23. **Rook, A.,** Plant dermatitis in general practice, *The Practitioner*, 188, 627, 1962.
24. **Lord, K. A. and Johnson, C. G.,** Production of dermatitis by pyrethrum and attempts to produce non-irritant extract, *Br. J. Dermat.*, 59, 367, 1947.

25. **Hjorth, N. and Fregert, S.,** Contact dermatitis in *Textbook of Dermatology,* Vol. I, Rook, A., Wilkinson, D. S., and Ebling, F. J. G., Eds., Blackwell Sci., Oxford, 1968, 288.
26. **Mitchell, J. C., Schofield, W. B., Singh, B. and Towers, G. H. N.,** Allergy to *Frullania, Arch. Derm.,* 100, 46, 1969.
27. **Mitchell, J. C., Fritig, B., Singh, B., and Towers, G. H. N.,** Allergic contact dermatitis from *frullania* and compositae. The role of sesquiterpens laetones, *J. Inv. Derm.,* 54, 233, 1970.
28. **Knoche, H., Ourisson, G., Perold, G. W., Foussereau, J., and Malevill, J.,** The allergenic component of a liverwort: a sesquiterpere lactone, *Science,* 166, 239, 1969.
29. **Mitchell, J. C. and Dupuis, G.,** Allergic contact dermatitis from sesquiterpenoids of the compositae family of plants, *Br. J. Derm.,* 84, 139, 1971.
30. **Mitchell, J. C.,** Stereoisomeric specificity of usnic acid in delayed hypersensitivity, *J. Inv. Derm.,* 47, 167, 1966.
31. **Rostenburg, A., Jr. and Good, C. K.,** Gaillardia dermatitis: hitherto unreported plant cause of dermatitis venenata, *JAMA,* 104, 1496, 1935.
32. **Pearlman, F.,** *Symposium on Foods — Proteins and Their Reactions,* Schulz, H. W., and Anglemier, H. F., Eds., AVI Publishing, Westport, Conn., 1964, 423.
33. **Strauss, M.,** Food allergens in *Proteins and Their Reactions,* Schulz, H. W. and Anglemier, H. F., Eds., AVI Publishing, Westport, Conn., 1964, 409.
34. **Strauss, M. B. and Spain, W. C.,** Preparation of active allergenic extracts: method of prevention of pigmentary oxidative products *J. Allergy,* 12, 61, 1940.
35. **Pearlman, F.,** Allergens in *Toxic Constituents of Plant Foodstuffs,* Liener, I. E., Ed., Academic Press, New York, 1969.
36. **Allen, P. Z. and Kabat, E. A.,** Studies on the capacity of some polysaccharides to elicit antibody formation in man, *J. Exp. Med.,* 105, 383, 1957.
37. **Griepetrog, Von F.,** Allergy studies with simple chemical compounds. VII. Nordihydroquaiaretic acid, *Arzneim. Forsch.,* 11, 920, 1961.
38. **Freedman, S. O., Siddiqui, A. I., Krupey, J. H., and Sehon, A. H.,** Identification of a simple chemical compound (chlorogenic acid) as an in plant materials causing human atopic diseases, *Am. J. Med. Sci.,* 244, 548, 1962.
39. **Randolph, T. G.,** Chemical contaminants of foods, *The 19th Series of Intern. Correspondence Soc. Allergists,* Columbus, Ohio, 1956.
40. **Walzer, M.,** Studies in absorption of undigested proteins in human beings. I. A simple direct method of studies of the absorption of undigested protein, *J. Immunol.,* 14, 143, 1929.
41. **Malkin, J. I. and Markow, M.,** An analysis of the comparative results of skin testing with cooked and uncooked foods, *J. Allergy,* 10, 337, 1952.
42. **Saperstein, S. and Anderson, D. W.,** Antigenicity of milk proteins of prepared formulas measured by precipitin ring test and passive cutaneous anaphylaxis in the guinea pig, *J. Pediatrics,* 61, 196, 1962.
43. **Vaughan, W. T. and Black, J. H.,** *Practice of Allergy,* C. V. Mosby Co., St. Louis, 1948.
44. **Baldwin, H. S. and Benedict, M. I.,** Mutual absorption tests with related foods, *J. Allergy,* 8, 120, 1937.
45. **Withers, O. R.,** Food allergens: A statistical analysis of 43 cases relative to genetic classifications of foods, *South. Med. J.,* 30, 918, 1937.
46. **Tuft, L. and Blumstein, G. I.,** Studies in food allergy. II. Sensitization to fresh fruits — clinical and experimental observations. *J. Allergy,* 13, 572, 1955.
47. **Tuft, L., Ettelson, L. N., and Schwartz, H.,** Allergy to foods containing sulfur amino acids, especially methionine: a case report and clinical study, *Am. J. Med. Sci.,* 229, 26, 1955.
48. **Matsumura, T., Tateno, K., Yugami, S., and Kuroumi, T.,** Six cases of buckwheat asthma induced by buckwheat flour attached to buckwheat chaff in pillows, *J. Asthma Res.,* 1, 219, 1964.
49. **Lamson, R. W.,** Sudden death associated with the injection of foreign substance, *J. Am. Med. Assoc.,* 82, 1091, 1924.
50. **Layton, L. L., Lee, S., Yamanaka, E., Greene, F. C., and Green, T. W.,** Allergy skin test upon castor-bean-sensitive humans and passively sensitized cynomolgus monkey, *Intern. Arch. Allergy Appl. Immunol.,* 20, 257, 1961.
51. **Perlman, F.,** Food allergy and vegetable proteins, *Food Technol. (Chicago),* 20, 1438, 1966.
52. **Ratner, B., Utrecht, S., Crawford, L. V., Malone, H. J., and Retsina, M.,** Allergenicity of modified and processed foodstuffs. V. Soybean. Influence of heat on its allergenicity. Use of soybean preparation for milk substitute, *Am. J. Dis. Child.,* 89, 187, 1955.
53. **Fries, J. H.,** Experience with allergy to soybean in the United States, *J. Asthma Res.,* 3, 209, 1966.
54. **Hale, R.,** Seeds as a source of food testing material, *Ann. Allergy,* 18, 270, 1960.
55. **Pearlman, F.,** Allergenic extracts — a comparison of their quality and reliability, *J. Allergy,* 30, 24, 1959.
56. **Fries, J. H., and Glazer, I.,** Studies in antigenicity of banana, raw and dehydrated, *J. Allergy,* 21, 169, 1950.

57. **Harris, M. C. and Shure, N.,** Sudden death due to allergy tests, *J. Allergy,* 21, 208, 1950.
58. **Spies, J. R.,** The chemistry of Allergen. XIX. On the number of antigens and the homogenicity of the isolated antigens of factors C.B.I.A. from castorbeans, *Ann. Allergy,* 25, 29, 1967.
59. **Fries, J. H.,** The cocoa bean and the allergic child, *Ann. Allergy,* 24, 484, 1966.
60. **Layton, L. L. and Yamanaka, E.,** Demonstrations of human reagins to foods, cat dander, an insect, and ragweed and grass pollens, *J. Allergy,* 33, 271, 1962.
61. **Girard, J. P., Rose, N. R., Kurz, M. L., Kobayashi, S., and Arbesman, C.,** *In vitro* lymphocyte transformation in atopic patients induced by antigens, *J. Allergy,* 39, 65, 1967.
62. **Bluminк, E.,** Food allergy. The chemical nature of substances eliciting symptoms, *World Rev. Nutr.,* 12, 505, 1970.
63. **Pearlman, F. and Layton, L. L.,** Stability and behavior of reaginic antibodies. Effects of freezing, thawing and lyophilizing on skin sensitizing activity of reaginic sera, *J. Allergy,* 39, 205, 1967.
64. **Rowe, A. H.,** Food allergy. Reasons for delayed recognition and control by physicians, *Q. Rev. Allergy Appl. Immunol.,* 8, 391, 1954.
65. **Goldman, A. S., Anderson, D. W., Jr., Sellers, W. A., and Saperstein, S.,** Milk allergy: I. Oral challenge with milk and isolated milk proteins in allergic children, *Pediatrics,* 32, 425, 1963.
66. **Ancona, G. R. and Schumacher, I. C.,** Frozen raw foods as skin testing materials. Further studies of use in cases of allergic disorders, *Calif. Med.,* 80, 181, 1954.
67. **Josephson, B. M. and Glaser, J.,** A comparison of skin testing with natural foods and commercial extracts, *Ann. Allergy,* 21, 33, 1963.
68. **Shelley, W. B.,** Methods of observing basophil leucocyte degranulation response, *Ann. N.Y. Acad. Sci.,* 103, 427, 1963.
69. **Levy, D. A. and Osler, A. G.,** Studies on the mechanism of hypersensitivity phenomenon. XIV; Passive sensitization *in vitro* of human leucocytes to ragweed pollen antigen, *J. Immunol.,* 97, 203, 1966.
70. **Layton, L. L., Dante, B. T., Moss, L. K., Dye, N. H., and DeEds, F.,** Electrophoretic fractionation of soluble antigenic proteins from the seeds of *Ricinus communis* (castor bean), *J. Am. Oil Chemists' Soc.,* 38, 405, 1961.
71. **Witten, V. H. and Shair, H. M.,** Repeated patch testing in allergic eczematons sensitization, *Ann. Allergy,* 7, 32, 1949.
72. **Slater, B. J., Norris, J. L., and Francis, N.,** Ragweed dermatitis: therapy by oral route, *Ann. Allergy,* 6, 594, 1948.
73. **Sulzberger, M. B. and Wise, F.,** Ragweed dermatitis with sensitization and desensitization phenomena, *JAMA,* 94, 93, 1930.
74. **Becker, S. W. and O'Brien, M. P.,** Value of patch tests in Dermatology, *Arch. Derm.,* 79, 569, 1959.
75. **Dorsey, C. S.,** Plant dermatitis in California, *Calif. Med.,* 96, 12, 1962.
76. **Robertson, W. D. and Mitchell, J. C.,** Allergic contact and photodermatitis, *Can. Med. Ass.,* 97, 380, 1967.
77. **Moslein, P.,** Pflanzen als Kontakt-allergene, *Berufskermatosen,* 11, 24, 1963.
78. **Balyeat, R. M., Rinkel, H. J., and Stemen, T. R.,** Contact dermatitis (venenata). Distribution and importance of the Heleniums as a cause of contact dermatitis in the United States, *Am. J. Med. Sci.,* 184, 547, 1932.
79. **McCord, C. P.,** The occupational toxicity of cultivated flowers, *Indust. Med. and Surg.,* 31, 365, 1962.
80. **O'Quinn, S. E. and Isbell, K. H.,** Influence of oral prednisone on eczematous patch test reactions, *Arch. Derm.,* 99, 380, 1969.
81. **Schwarz, L. and Warren, L. H.,** Dermatitis caused by contact with copperweed (*Oxytemia acerosa*), *J. Allergy,* 12, 63, 1940.
82. **Smith, L. M. and Hughes, R. P.,** Dermatitis caused by Mexican rubber plant, *Arch. Derm. Syph.,* 38, 780, 1938.
83. **Hand, E. A.,** Contact dermatitis due to cape weed, *Arch. Dermat. and Syph.,* 49, 331, 1944.
84. **Woods, B.,** Irritant plants, *Trans. St. John's Hosp. Dermat. Soc.,* (new series) 48, 75, 1962.
85. **McCord, C. P., Kilker, C. H., and Minister, D. K.,** Pyrethrum dermatitis. A record of the occurrence of occupational dermatoses among workers in the pyrethrum industry, *JAMA,* 77, 448, 1921.
86. **Schwartz, L., Tulipan, L., and Birmingham, D. J.,** *Occupational diseases of the skin,* 3rd ed., Lea and Febiger, Philadelphia, 1957, 650.
87. **Janke, D., Durch Lowenzahn** (*Taraxacum officinale*) verursachtes ekzem, *Hautarzt,* 1, 177, 1950.
88. **Brunsting, L. and Anderson, C. R.,** Ragweed dermatitis, *JAMA,* 103, 1285, 1934.

Chapter 12

IONIZING RADIATION EFFECTS ON THE IMMUNE RESPONSE SYSTEM

S. G. Oberg and R. P. Sharma

TABLE OF CONTENTS

I. INTRODUCTION

Since Murphy's[1] utilization of radiation to interfere with lymphocyte function in order to modify tumor transplant rejection rates in 1914, many researchers have investigated the relationship between the application of ionizing radiations and subsequent alterations of the immune response system in mammals. Excellent literature reviews by Taliaferro et al. in 1951,[2] and again in their monograph of 1964,[3] represent thorough evaluations of works conducted since the immunosuppressive effects of radiation were first recognized early in the century. Intense research in the area has continued during the last decade as modern instrumentation and refined laboratory techniques have evolved. Improved sensitivity in the areas of radiation quality evaluation, cell separation procedures, and biochemical identification of cellular subpopulations continues to foster appreciation among immunologists and radiobiologists for the complexity of the radiation-effected alterations of the antigen-antibody relationship.

The purpose of this chapter, rather than to provide a comprehensive literature review on the subject of radiation immunology, is to present some selected published efforts in the field that represent the status of projects that deal with further elucidation of immune mechanisms. Particularly it is intended that ionizing radiation should be appreciated as an otherwise toxic agent that, under controlled situations, finds positive applications in both laboratory research (i.e., as an adjunct tool in delineating the basic mechanisms of immune reactions), and in specific clinical applications (such as in the modification of graft vs. host tissue reactions).

II. RADIATION TOXICITY

Virtually from the time of their discoveries, X-rays and gamma rays were known to cause adverse biological effects. Because of their promising futures in medical applications, however, investigators extensively studied the rays with the motive of optimizing their benefits while reducing harmful side effects. Through the ensuing years it was determined that ionizing radiations were able to yield diagnostic information and provide therapeutic advantages that were unobtainable by other methods. At the same time, when excessive radiation doses were unwittingly or accidently applied to laboratory and clinical subjects, it was learned that radiation caused no exotic or previously unheard of disease states. Radiation insults do have some unique toxicological properties such as specificity of effects on critical molecules of the nucleoplasm, the rapid rate at which biological damage occurs, and their ability to destroy the body's normal immune response mechanisms. In general, however, radiation injuries were seen to mimic the effects of other 'poisons' (that could be delivered to all parts of the body at once, have cumulative effects, and affect some body tissues more than others), so it became reasonable to discuss ionizing radiation as physical phenomena that could be overtly toxic when 'taken' in excess.

Scientists continue to debate the limits of so-called safe doses of radiation. Traditionally organizations, such as the National Council on Radiation Protection and Measurements, that recommend safe working levels of radiation in occupational situations have subscribed to the hypothesis that for any absorbed radiation dose there would be a proportional biologic response (the linear or nonthreshold theory). At lower dose levels (near natural background quantities) the limits were considered to be conservative[4] due to the difficulty in actually determining alterations in most measurable biologic endpoints.

III. TOTAL DOSE AND DOSE-RATE EFFECTS

Recently Sternglass[5] evaluated low dose and low dose rate effects on cell membranes and has implicated small radiation insults with damage to bone marrow cells and reduced antibody responses. His thesis is that at low dose rates, below 10^{-3} rad/min, the production of highly reactive free radicals (O_2^-) in cell fluids causes increases in cell membrane permeability. He has reported that this effect is more predominant than direct radiation 'hits' on critical intracellular structures. Furthermore, he suggested that low dose rates and less densely ionizing radiations aggravate the condition because the opportunity for free radicals to recombine is lessened. A corollary observation is that high linear energy transfer radiations such as alpha and other heavy particles are much less efficient in producing free radicals than are the lower linear energy transfer type of ionizing radiations such as X-rays and gamma rays, and are responsible for a high proportion of direct radiation effects.

The high toxicity of O_2^- free radicals is apparently due to their ability to initiate oxidative chain reactions in phospholipid membranes and, according to Sternglass, the radiations that produce low ion densities (increased production of O_2^-) may be 100 to 1000 times more damaging than expected from high dose rate experimental results. Because membrane damage is an indirect somatic effect, Sternglass feels that cell functions involved in immune protection may be compromised by exposure to low levels of man made or natural environmental radiations.

Chaskes et al.[6] examined serum immunoglobulin levels in humans exposed to therapeutic levels of total body gamma irradiation. Their treatment regimen consisted of 10 R/day or 30 R/day exposures until doses of 100, 150, 200, or 250 R had been provided. As an additional variable, exposure delivery rates of 1.5 R/hr or 1.5 R/min were utilized. The authors determined that, considering 20% normal variability in their patients' immunoglobulin levels, most post-therapy levels were significantly lower than pretherapy values. Serum IgG levels were found to be the least affected by radiation while IgA appeared to be more sensitive to radiation-induced alteration than were IgM or IgG. Bazier and Malet[7] reported the same depression pattern in irradiated mice.

Because patients in the Chaskes study suffered from different forms of malignant disorders, and because the sample population was quite small, statistical treatment of the data was limited. It was noted by the authors, however, that the frequency and severity of immunoglobulin depression was greater with larger total doses. An unexpected finding, however, coincided with Sternglass' observations in that larger and more frequent immunoglobulin depressions followed the low dose rate exposure of 1.5 R/hr. The sample size in this case, however, was too small for vigorous statistical verification.

Carlson and Gengozian[8] examined the radiation exposure rate dependence of the immune response in mice and determined that antibody formation decreased as the exposure rate increased. Their studies featured gamma ray treatments from ^{60}Co at exposure rates of 8, 40, and 72 R/min before or after challenges with rat or sheep erythrocytes. The authors compared antibody formation suppression curves with mortality data and concluded that exposure rate sensitivity between 8 and 40 R/min was greater for immune suppression than for 30 day mortality, while mortality was more rate-dependent than immune suppression at exposure rates between 40 and 72 R/min. A later report[9] confirmed these findings and in 1971, Carlson and Lubet[10] reported that the activity of both T and B cells was sensitive to differences in dose rate between 8-80 rads/min. In particular, it was noted that B cell function appeared to be significantly more dose-rate dependent when compared to residual activity of T cells.

Gottleib and Gengozian[11] exposed mice to X-rays (7.6-67 rads/min) or fission spectrum neutrons (2.8-93 rads/min) and found dose rate dependence for X-ray exposures but not for the high LET (linear energy transfer) neutron treatments. Injections of sheep erythrocytes shortly after X-irradiation showed that the extent of immunosuppression was a function of both total dose and dose rate, whereas only total dose appeared to be a factor following neutron exposures. Quantifying these relationships further, the authors reported[12] that the magnitude of the dose rate effect was an experimental function of the linear energy transfer value of the radiation, and there also existed an inverse cube root dose-rate relationship.

Specific evaluation of graft vs. host (GVH) reactivity in mice was considered by Hayakawa and Tsuchiya[13] as a function of radiation dose rate (chronic vs. acute). They observed that although spleen size was reduced in continuously irradiated mice, the GVH reactivity on a per cell basis was less when compared to the acutely exposed mice (at the 600 R level).

IV. RADIATION IMMUNOSUPPRESSION TECHNIQUES

To achieve an irradiation technique for the induction of transplantation tolerance that is both efficacious and safe to the human recipient has proven to be a difficult task for investigators (Table 1). When experimenting with laboratory animals the treatments employed require that: (1) the procedure should prove relatively safe for humans, (2) the techniques should be applicable to outbred species, and (3) long term survival of allogeneic organ grafts must be achieved.[14]

Chanana et al.[15] list several methods utilized to selectively induce immunosuppression by radiation as: (1) surface radiation applicators for individual lymphoid organs, (2) irradiation of individual lymphoid organs such as the thymus and the spleen, (3) irradiation of allografts immediately following transplantation or during rejection episodes, (4) indwelling intravascular radiation sources, (5) intravascular or intralymphatic injection of radioisotopes, and (6) extracorporeal irradiation of blood or lymph. Other variations of these procedures would be total lymphoid irradiation,[14,16] transfusions with irradiated blood[17,18] and various schemes of single whole body exposure or continuous low level irradiation supported with bone marrow reconstitution.[13]

Using extracorporeal irradiation of blood (ECIB) and extracorporeal irradiation of lymph (ECIL), Chanana's group found that they could produce lymphocytopenia in the blood and lymph, and also cause depletion of lymphocytes in the lymphoreticular organs. In the case of ECIB, blood is routed near a ^{137}Cs source via cartoid jugular shunts (thoracic duct-jugular vein shunts are used for ECIL). When blood was allowed to circulate near the gamma source for the equivalent of 5 blood volumes, it was determined that most of the blood lymphocytes received about 500 rads. Because radiosensitivity of erythrocytes was not a factor, ECIL was performed at about 1000 rads.

Through various experimental procedures the authors determined that: (1) lymphocytes passing through the irradiator were so damaged that they were unable to home on the lymph nodes, proliferate, and return to the thoracic duct, (2) lymphocytopenia induced by ECIB and ECIL is the result of radiation injury to circulating lymphocytes and is not mediated by corticosteroid hormones, (3) the combination of thymectomy and ECIB is no more effective in prolonging skin allograft survival than is ECIB alone, and (4) ECIB and azathioprine apparently have synergistic immunosuppressive effects on skin allografts. Following clinical trials of human renal transplants, the investigators further concluded that recipients treated by ECIB had fewer and less severe acute rejection episodes, and renal function and graft survival were better than in the nonECIB treated group. Additionally, although extracorporeal irradiation effectively eliminates

Table 1
SELECTED ILLUSTRATIONS OF IRRADIATION TECHNIQUES IN DIFFERENT ANIMAL SPECIES AND ASSOCIATED IMMUNOLOGIC EFFECTS

Technique	Dose	Species	Results	Ref.
Extracorporeal Irradiation of Blood (ECIB)	15-60 rad transit dose	Cattle	Slightly prolonged survival of skin allografts	51
Extracorporeal Irradiation of Lymph (ECIL)	800-2000 rad transit dose	Cattle		52 15
Local kidney graft irradiation	600 rads total (150 rads each on alternate days in first post-transplant week)	Humans	Promoted transplant acceptance	53
Topical x-irradiation to heart transplants	2400 rads total (400 rads twice weekly from first post-operative day)	Dogs	Prolonged allograft survival	54
Endolymphatic irradiation with ^{198}Au and ^{32}P	35,000 rads to lymph nodes (^{198}Au); 150,000 rads to lymph nodes (^{32}P)	Humans	Temporary effect on immune response; little practical application in kidney transplants	20
Continuous ^{32}P irradiation of spleen	97,000 rads	Rats	Lymphopenia via killing of small recirculating lymphocytes	55 56
Continuous ^{32}P irradiation of appendix	150,000 rads	Rabbits	Lymphopenia produced without advantage to skin graft survival	57
Blood replacement from irradiated donors	1600 rads to donors	Sheep	Various granulocyte changes; decrease in number of immature myeloid elements in bone marrow	17 18
Fractionated total lymphoid irradiation	3400 rads (200 rads/day, 5 times per week)	Mice	Prolonged skin and bone allograft survival	14 16
Regional lymph node irradiation	2300 rads (in 5 equal fractions given on alternate days following sensitization)	Rats	Both cellular and humoral immune responses acutely and markedly depressed	58

the body's mobile pool of lymphocytes, it is less efficient at depleting more sessile members which contain immunocompetent cells.

Fuks et al.[19] have described a radiotherapy regimen of fractionated total lymphoid irradiation (TLI), used in the treatment of human malignant lymphomas, that appears to produce few undesirable side effects. These techniques when used in the treatment of Hodgkin's disease prove to be quite immunosuppressive by eliminating the mixed leukocyte reaction for 2-3 years and by inducing T-lymphocytopenia that persists for at least 10 years in man. In their studies with TLI on mice,[14,16] where body parts other than lymphoid organs are shielded from radiation, the same group has shown that rejection of skin allografts can be impaired and that chimerism after infusion of semi-allogeneic bone marrow cells occurs for at least 6 months. The authors hypothesize, based on their observation that lymphocyte repopulation patterns are permanently altered following TLI, the TLI not only depletes lymphocytes, but also alters the reticular and endothelial structure of the lymphoid tissues to the extent that maturation, homing and T-lymphocyte interactions may be permanently disturbed. These findings may be clinically significant in that the procedure is safe in humans, donors and recipients can be allogeneic, and in test situations with mice, bone marrow and skin graft survival appeared to be permanent.

As an example of the technique involving intralymphatic injection of radioisotopes, the study of Birkeland et al.[20] is cited. In this case endolymphatic irradiation with ^{198}Au and ^{32}P was employed in an attempt to produce immunosuppression in renal transplant situations. Data were obtained from 12 patients injected with ^{198}Au and 8 patients with ^{32}P. The isotopes were injected, in volumes of 0.5 mℓ, into lymph vessels on the dorsal side of the foot and the radioisotope progress and localization was determined with gamma cameras.

Calculations indicated that the dose to the blood was only about 0.1 rad, to tissues about 6-7 cm from the lymph nodes the dose was about 20 rads, while the dose to lymph nodes was as much as 35,000 rads from ^{198}Au or 150,000 rads from ^{32}P. Immunosuppressive effects were observed in these clinical trials, however, most effects appeared to be quite transient and the authors conclude that the potential risk of side effects overrides the possible advantage of using the method routinely in transplant situations.

Souto and Anderson[17] assessed the effects of substituting blood of normal sheep with that from other normal sheep, from sheep in which leukocytes had been removed mechanically, and from sheep that had experienced whole body irradiations of 1,600 R by ^{60}Co. They found that regeneration of granulocytes, observed in the peripheral blood, occurred after 16 months in the irradiated-to-normal transfusions, whereas regeneration was witnessed after 8 weeks in the other test subjects.

In a corollary study[18] the same authors evaluated cell distributions in bone marrow of animals whose blood was replaced with that from lethally irradiated donors and found: (1) decreases in the number of immature myeloid elements, (2) increases in the numbers of immature erythroid cells, and (3) decreases in the immature myeloid/erythroblast ratio.

Using radiation exposure regimens of 600 R acute, 1800 R chronic (5 R/day for 1 year), and bone marrow reconstitution after 600 R acute, Hayakawa and Tsuchiya[13] examined the causes of long-term radiation effects on graft vs. host reactions in mice. They found that after 1 year the graft vs. host reactivity of the spleen was impaired after acute and chronic radiation exposures and that bone marrow transplantation did not prevent that impairment of reactivity. The 600 R acute exposure appeared to have the greater effect on reactivity per cell and this dose affected the reactivity decline more severely than could be accounted for by advancing age of the mice alone. In comparing their results with Nelson et al.,[21] Hayakawa and Tsuchiya express suspicion that the long term impairment of graft vs. host reactivity after 600 R of acute radiation was not due to defects intrinsic to the cells but rather to extrinsic defects, such as a failure of a regulatory factor to support the successful maturation and proliferation of cells.

V. RADIATION-INDUCED IMMUNOLOGIC ALTERATION AND SENSITIVITY TO LEUKEMIA

The presence and release of leukemogenic agents in irradiated nonleukemic tissues for a brief period of time following fractionated irradiation was reported in 1966.[22] The correlation between radiation induced immunosuppression and radiogenic leukemia is an interesting aspect of radiobiology that offers a different perspective on the complex role of radiation "toxicity" with regard to the immune response system. Haran-Ghera[23] attempted to further evaluate the agent release phenomena by isolating leukemogenic filtrates from normal tissues of young and old mice. Considerations of time limitations and types of tissue involvement led the author to postulate that a possible contributing factor in the process was the transient depression of immunological responsiveness induced by irradiation. In another report[24] Haran-Ghera established that the rate of lymphoma development was related to the x-ray dosage received by the host; induction began at 250-300 R and was maximally effective in mice at 550 R whole body exposure. This dose coincided with increased cellular immunity impairment and implicated the effect in facilitating neoplastic proliferation.

Clapp and Yuhas[25] confirmed that radiation not only induces malignant transformation, but it also reduces the ability of the host to resist the growth of the transformed clones. More specifically, Peled and Haran-Ghera[26] implicated thymus–derived cells in the mechanism allowing expression of the immunosuppressive effects of radiation leukemia viruses — the effect was not revealed with bone marrow derived populations of immunocytes.

Although the ability of radiation to induce leukemia was not doubted, Ihle et al.[27] were unable to relate leukemia incidence rates to the length of time that immune responses were activated. By utilizing endogenous ecotropic murine leukemia viruses and by recording the development of thymic lymphomas, the authors determined that incidence rates were comparable in mice that developed no immune response, developed transient immune responses, or developed persistant immune responses. An additional result of the experiments performed was that neither radiation-induced leukemia nor its suppression by bone marrow reconstitution can be credited to their influence on the humoral immune response to the virus.

VI. RADIATION EXPOSURE AND INFECTIVITY

Taliaferro et al.[3] have reviewed representative radiation induced changes in immune responses during the course of infections. Irradiation effects on the host-parasite relationship are variable because either (or both) the host or the parasite may be injured by the treatment. In many cases it is clear that parasite counts and reproductive activity are inversely related to the body's antibody forming ability, i.e., parasitic success follows immune suppression.

As might be suspected in post irradiation situations, the host animal reveals an increased susceptibility to infection during the period of depressed immunity.[28] Besides the impairment in antibody production ability, it has also been shown that macrophage incapacitation by radiation can allow bacteria to attain higher than control values.[29] In addition to decreases in the number of macrophages and their loss of digestive activity, radiation seems also to depress the action of specific serum bactericidins thus promoting susceptibility to particular kinds of infectious agents.[30]

Some infectious courses altered by radiation are not due to immunosuppressive actions per se. Singer[31] reported lower parasitemia (*Plasmodium berghei*) in mice injected 20 min prior to 550 R x-ray exposures. In this case the lower parasite populations were correlated with existing numbers of immature erythrocytes (hosts) which became depleted in time as a result of hemopoietic injury from the x-ray treatments. Occasionally radiation effects on the host immune response system can be beneficial. Hotchin and Weigand[32] considered mice infected with lymphocytic choriomeningitis and found that postinfection survival increased with X-ray doses after correction for X-ray death. Since animals are generally more radiosensitive than their parasites, however, cases of this type are somewhat unusual.

VII. EFFECT OF RADIATION ON IMMUNOCYTES

That lymphocytes are the principal cells involved in immune reactions has been known for many years. It has also been recognized that there are two major classes of lymphocytes that participate in immunologic situations and they have been called T cells, which require the thymus gland for development, and B cells, which develop independently of the thymus. In general, T cells appear to be responsible for cell mediated immunity, while B cells are primarily involved in humoral antibody responses.

When B cells are activated by antigen they divide and differentiate into blast cells with abundant endoplasmic reticulum and some go on to become plasma cells. These cells generally remain in the lymphoid tissue where they secrete large amounts of antibody which circulates in the blood. When T cells are activated by antigen, they proliferate and differentiate to become blast cells but do not develop large amounts of endoplasmic reticulum and do not become antibody secreting cells. They do, however, help B cells make antibody responses.[33]

Because resting T and B lymphocytes are morphologically indistinguishable and are found together in all peripheral lymphoid tissue, various techniques have been employed to differentially characterize the cells. Some methods devised to identify the cell types depend upon the ability of certain drugs and chemicals to preferentially deplete or stimulate one of the cell types. For example, phytohemagglutinin (PHA) appears to stimulate T cells primarily, while pokeweed mitogen (PWM) stimulates predominately B cells.[34,35] Variable radiation sensitivity also discriminates lymphocyte types and this sensitivity is of special interest to radiotherapists and clinicians involved in organ transplant situations.

Although differences in lymphocyte radiosensitivity are readily shown, it is not unequivocal as to which cell species displays the greater radiation effect (see Table 2). In human studies for example, Facchini et al.[36] determined greater T cell radiosensitivity in normal persons whose lymphocytes were exposed to ^{60}Co gamma rays in vitro. Their conclusions were based on electron microscopic determinations of membrane receptor alterations. Reddy et al.[37] also claimed greater absolute T cell radiosensitivity in adults whose thymic glands were irradiated in infancy. Percentage wise, Fuks et al.[19] found T cell decreases and Ig-bearing cell increases in patients formerly treated radiotherapeutically for Hodgkin's disease. Women exposed regionally to ^{60}Co gamma rays for treatment of mammary carcinomas revealed selective T lymphocyte lymphopenia,[38] and Byfield et al.[39] claimed B lymphocytes to be slightly less radiosensitive than T cells in patients who received mediastinal or pelvic radiotherapy treatments. Han et al. [40] examined cultured human lymphocytes and found that following in vitro exposures of 250

Table 2
STUDIES INVOLVING EXPOSURES TO RADIATION AND ITS EFFECTS ON VARIOUS IMMUNOLOGIC SITES OR FUNCTIONS

Effects observed and conclusions	Species	Irradiation	Technique	Ref.
T cells were found to be more radiosensitive than B cells	Normal humans	*In vitro* exposure of lymphocytes to ^{60}Co gamma rays (50-2500 rads)	Examination by electron microscopy of separated B and T cells revealed that lymphocyte membrane receptors behave differentially after exposure to radiation; radiation damage alters structural arrangement of chromatin	36
T cells show greater absolute radiosensitivity than B cells	Human adults	Thymic x-irradiation in infancy (270-564 R)	Absolute and relative numbers and mitotic activity of stimulated lymphocytes were determined and compared to normal donors	37
At moderate radiation doses, residual B cell activity was more suppressed than T cell activity	Male CD_2F_1 mice	Sub-lethal whole body irradiation to ^{60}Co gamma rays (200-950 rads at 8 or 80 rads/min)	Number of plaque forming cells/spleen were determined before and after reconstitution and antigenic challenges (SRBC); B cell function appeared to be dose-rate dependent	10
Patients in complete remission exhibited T-lymphocytopenia, B lymphocytosis, and increases of null lymphocytes; percentage of T cells was very low while the percentage of Ig bearing cells was significantly increased	Humans in complete remission from Hodgkin's Disease	Radiotherapy doses from 6 MeV linear accelerator (LINAC) in local, extended field, or total lymphoid irradiation modes	Lymphocytes were separated on a Ficoll-Hypaque gradient, identified and enumerated; also recorded were the mixed leukocyte reaction, stimulation of lymphocytes by PHA and Con A, and the degree of delayed hypersensitivity to dinitrochlorobenzene (DNCB)	19
B_γ lymphocytes are extremely sensitive to radiation while T cells consist of one subpopulation that is fairly radiosensitive and one (approximately 8%) that is extremely radioresistant	Male C3Hf/HeMs mice	Whole body exposures to ^{137}Cs gamma rays (47-10,000 R)	Fluorescent antibody stains of cell suspensions were performed; locations, disappearance kinetics, and survival curves for T and B lymphocytes in spleens were deduced with fluorescence microscopes	41

Table 2 (continued)
STUDIES INVOLVING EXPOSURES TO RADIATION AND ITS EFFECTS ON VARIOUS IMMUNOLOGIC SITES OR FUNCTIONS

Effects observed and conclusions	Species	Irradiation	Technique	Ref.
Circulating B lymphocytes may be slightly less radiosensitive than T, but both are depleted by customary doses of local radiotherapy for cancer	Human radiotherapy patients	Mediastinal or pelvic doses from therapy sources (2000-3000 rads total)	Total lymphocyte numbers, SRBC rosette forming ability, and ^{3}H-thymidine incorporation in response to PHA and pokeweed mitogen stimulation were measured	39
Parasternal irradiation for mammary carcinoma leads to long lasting lymphopenia which mainly is a selective T-lymphocyte lymphopenia	Adult women	^{60}Co gamma ray exposures to chest areas; (4200-4500 rads in therapy fractions)	Lymphocyte separations (Ficoll-Isopaque), transformation tests (PHA stimulation), SRBC rosette formation rates, extent of induced lymphopenia, and B/T cell ratios in peripheral blood were measured	38
The helper function of carrier-primed T cells was found to be radiosensitive *in vivo;* the results could not be attributed to interference with the spleen seeking properties of the irradiated cells	Highly inbred strains of mice	*In vivo* and *in vitro* exposures to x-irradiation (0-5000 rads)	Proliferative capacity of thoracic duct lymphocytes transferred to lethally irradiated mice, distribution of labeled thoracic duct derived lymphocytes irradiated *in vitro,* and effects on antihapten antibody responses were studied	42
Cultured T lymphoid cells are extremely radiosensitive and B lymphoid cells are fairly radioresistant (at 250 R, viable T cells were reduced by 95-100%, whereas only 2-7% of B cells were killed at day 1-4 of incubation)	Humans	*In vitro* exposures (100-4000 R)	Growth patterns of irradiated T & B cells were compared by ^{3}H-thymidine incorporation methods and viability tests	40
Cell mediated immune reaction (macrophage migration inhibition) can be detected after *in vitro* irradiation with moderately high doses (up to 10,000 rads), but it is significantly reduced with 5000 rads	Albino guinea pigs of both sexes	*In vitro* exposure to cell suspensions with ^{60}Co gamma rays (500 or 10,000 rads)	Migration rates of peritoneal cells from animals previously immunized with egg albumin were recorded	59

Supralethal doses of x-rays cause differential decreases in the serum levels of the Ig classes; the serum IgA level is related to the integrity of the gut epithelium and decreases in IgA may indicate x-ray-caused intestinal lesions	6 mo. old female hybrid mice	Whole body exposure to 260 kVp x-rays (1000-5000 R)	Serum concentrations of each Ig class was determined following various radiation doses	7
Irradiation-induced immunosuppression may be due to the suppression of formation rather than to destruction of cytotoxic effector cells	Male Sprague-Dawley rats and male C57B1 mice	*In vitro* exposure of cells to 250 kVp x-rays (0-2000 rads)	PHA response was determined, autoradiography was performed to trace the fate of PHA-induced blast cells, and cytolytic activity was studied	60
Lymph node germinal centers destroyed by radiation do not prevent formation of antibodies, therefore germinal center cells may be more involved with generation of memory cells than with antibody synthesis	Adult female swiss albino mice	Whole body exposures to ^{60}Co gamma rays (0-800 rads)	Effects of antigen form on radiosensitivity of primary and secondary antitoxin responses, immunogenicity of antigen-antibody complexes, and temporal effects of antigen booster injections were analyzed	61
Clonogenic survival in spleens of irradiated mice indicated that late radiation effects may be due to factors other than cellular proliferation of vital stromal cells	2½ - 3 mo. old male C3H/HeJ mice	Spleens exposed *in vivo* to 250 kVp x-rays (500-3000 rads); additional mice exposed whole body	The ability of irradiated spleens or bone marrow to support clonal proliferation of hematopoietic stem cells was determined as a function of total dose, dose fractionation and time of measurement after irradiation	21
Two forms of progenitor cells (different degrees of radiosensitivity) were determined in diffusion chamber studies of murine hematopoeitic stem cells	Male (C_3H × DBA/2) hybrid mice and female randomly bred mice	Whole body exposures to 250 kVp x-rays (hosts received two 300 rad doses)	Bone marrow cells were implanted in the abdomens of hosts; upon sacrifice, differential cell counts were made and cells were identified as proliferative or nonproliferative granulocytes or macrophages	49
A prerequisite for B-T cell interactions involving irradiated T cells is the differentiation of bone marrow derived precursor cells in the spleens of irradiated mice	6-12 wk. old female mice (BALB/c × DBA/2)F_1	Recipients exposed to whole body exposures to ^{137}Cs gamma rays (1000 rads); cell suspensions exposed *in vitro*	Frequencies of anti-SRBC response in spleens of irradiated mice reconstituted with thymus-derived cells, marrow-derived cells, or cell mixtures were recorded along with responses subsequent to reconstitution with irradiated T cells and nonirradiated T cells and nonirradiated B cells	50

Table 2 (continued)
STUDIES INVOLVING EXPOSURES TO RADIATION AND ITS EFFECTS ON VARIOUS IMMUNOLOGIC SITES OR FUNCTIONS

Effects observed and conclusions	Species	Irradiation	Technique	Ref.
Irradiation suppresses mitoses and is most effective in embryonic stages when the mitotic index is highest. Regeneration of thymic cells in irradiated embryos appears to recapitulate normal embryology as the latter recapitulates phylogeny	Pouch young "embryo" opossums varying from 1-50 days of postnatal age	Embryos attached to maternal tissue were exposed to 384 rads of 250 kVp x-rays (mothers and embryos were shielded by lead)	Thymus size was noted and size distribution of lymphocytes was recorded; the mitotic index, Hassall's corpuscles, and regeneration rates were examined	62
Stem cells flow from one marrow to the other and, if the regulatory barrier for division in one marrow is weakened by irradiation, immigrant cells settle and proliferate there	2 mo. old male CBA/H and CBA/H-T_6T_6 mice	Whole body exposures to 250 kVp x-rays (400 R), or right hind leg only exposures to 800 R	Proliferative capacity of chromosomally marked bone marrow or spleen cells was recorded after injection into sublethally irradiated mice	63
Cells of the cell-bound type of immunity undergo their immunologic maturation within the thymus and are subsequently seeded into other lymphoid organs	1 mo. old (A.CA × C57BL) F_1-hybrid mice	Whole body exposures to 200 kVp x-rays (800 R)	Recovery of the hemolysin-response against SRBC after lethal irradiation and bone marrow reconstitution in mice was studied	46
Source of T cells is not thymic elements but is from hemopoeitic precursors — progenitors differentiate in the thymus; T cell precursors are more abundant in bone marrow than in adult spleen and are absent from peripheral lymph nodes	5-6 wk old female mice (AKR/J, AKR/T, and AKR/C)	Whole body exposures to ^{137}Cs gamma rays (760 R)	Inhibition of ^{3}H-thymidine incorporation by specific antisera was assayed and the distribution of injected nucleated bone marrow cells was recorded	64
Thymic regeneration after lethal x-ray doses demonstrated the existence of a very radioresistant stem cell pool, possibly located in the thymus itself	12-20 wk old female A/J mice	Whole body exposures to ^{137}Cs gamma rays (760 R) or 280 kVp x-ray exposures with spleen and bone marrow shields	Cell counts, histopathology, antisera studies, and cytotic tests were performed during thymic regeneration phases	44

Optimal expression of GVH reactions may require the participation of at least 2 subpopulations of thymus derived cells	7-9 wk old mice of various strains	Whole body exposures to 200 kVp x-rays (800 R)	*In vivo* passage of normal spleen cells into irradiated syngeneic hosts was recorded; migratory patterns were related to cell reactivities, specificities, and sensitivities	43
The assumption that the thymus is seeded from bone marrow is not needed to explain a biphasic pattern of thymus regeneration, rather it is likely that cells present in the thymus or deposited there immediately after injection of bone marrow cells can engender a full regeneration of the thymus	12 wk old inbred strains of mice	Whole body exposures to 250 kVp x-rays (605 rads)	Irradiated animals, irradiated animals treated with bone marrow cells from normal AKR donors and irradiated animals treated with bone marrow cells from irradiated AKR donors were studied; mitotic index, thymus weight, and chromosome analysis was recorded for each specimen	48

R, viable T cell populations were reduced 95-100% whereas only 2-7% of B cells were killed.

Studies with mice tend to indicate similar relative radiosensitivities for the two lymphocyte populations but other factors have been found to influence experimental conclusions. In Carlson and Lubets' recent report[10] it was claimed that at moderate radiation doses (sublethal whole body gamma irradiation), residual B cell activity was more suppressed than T cell activity. Additionally, B cell function appeared to be dose rate dependent. Analyses of T and B cells in murine spleens led Kataoka and Sado[41] to report that B_γ lymphocytes are extremely radiosensitive while T cells consist of two subpopulations, one of which is fairly radiosensitive and one (approximately 8%) which is extremely radioresistant. Other authors have indicated multiple functions of T cells[42] or have isolated unique subpopulations among thymus–derived lymphocytes.[43]

The success or failure of therapeutic tissue transplants depends heavily upon the combined reactivities of T and B lymphocytes. Although immunosuppression by radiation has proven efficacious in various modalities there remains much to be learned about the actual mechanisms of such processes. Recovery of immunologic competence has been related to the status of the lymphoid organs — primarily the spleen, thymus, and bone marrow. Thymic restoration following irradiation may derive from an intrathymic resident pool of radioresistant stem cells. Kadish and Basch[44] found thymic regeneration rates were unaffected by injections of syngeneic bone marrow cells, or by bone marrow and spleen shielding during irradiation. In a later article[45] the authors indicated that thymic lymphocytes do not arise from endogenous thymic elements but are derived from hematopoietic precursors. These progenitor cells evidently enter the thymus by way of the blood stream.

In measuring degrees of immunologic competence recovery following irradiation, as affected by bone marrow reconstitution and antigenic challenges, Blomgren and Andersson[46] considered the influence of the thymus on immunologic maturation of the lymphoid system. Since they found the existence of a small pool of highly immunologically competent cells in the thymus,[47] they were later able to conclude that cells of the cell-bound type of immunity undergo their immunologic maturation within the thymus and are subsequently seeded into other lymphoid organs. Decleve et al.[48] recorded spleen and bone marrow cell division rates along with thymic regeneration parameters and deduced that cells present in the thymus, or deposited there immediately after injection of bone marrow cells, could engender full regeneration of the thymus. In evaluating only the inactivation of murine hematopoietic stem cells by irradiation, Petersen, Bøyun, and Laane[49] found unequal degrees of radiosensitivity between two different types of progenitor cells. And finally, Ito et al.[50] when examining the prerequisites of B-T cell interactions involving irradiated T cells, found evidence that differentiation of bone marrow-derived precursor cells outside the bone cavities (in the spleen of irradiated mice) was a necessary condition for functional interactions.

VIII. CONCLUSION

From the foregoing but brief review it is apparent that radiation produces a multitude of effects on the immunologic systems. In spite of the fact that the application of radiation has played a very important role in development of knowledge in the field of immunology and in elucidating the underlying cellular mechanisms, the exact nature of damage that radiation produces on immune response mechanisms is not fully understood. The discovery that there are numerous subpopulations of immunocompetent cells can be attributed largely to their radiation sensitivity. Similar to many other toxic agents, radiation can produce dose-dependent stimulation and depression on selected immunologic parameters. Low doses may sometimes enhance the immune responsiveness, whereas the moderate to high doses are often immunosuppressive to either the same or different processes.

That radiation exposure alters the host responsiveness to infections and can alter the immune surveillance that may be important in neoplastic survival, makes radiation-immunology an important field of investigation. It is particularly important since the exposure to some ionizing radiation is rather unavoidable even outside of the therapeutic situation. Further research is needed both in defining the specific effects of radiation on immune processes and how radiation-induced manipulation of such processes can modify the responsiveness of the organism to foreign substances.

REFERENCES

1. **Murphy, J. B.,** Heteroplastic tissue grafting effected through Roentgen-ray lymphoid destruction, *JAMA,* 62, 1459, 1914.
2. **Taliaferro, W. H. and Taliaferro, L. G.,** Effects of x-rays on immunity: a review, *J. Immunol.,* 66, 181, 1951.
3. **Taliaferro, W. H., Taliaferro, L. G., and Jaroslow, B. N.,** *Radiation and Immune Mechanisms,* Academic Press, New York, 1964.
4. **Russell, W. L., Russell, L. B., and Kelly, E. M.,** Radiation dose rate and mutation frequency, *Science,* 128, 1546, 1958.
5. **Sternglass, E. J.,** The role of indirect radiation effects on cell membranes in the immune response, in *Radiation and the Lymphatic System,* Ballou, J. E., Ed., ERDA Symp. Ser. 37, CONF-740930, National Technical Information Service, Springfield, Va., 185, 1976.
6. **Chaskes, S., Kingdon, G. C., and Balish, E.,** Serum immunoglobulin levels in humans exposed to therapeutic total-body gamma irradiation, *Radiat. Res.,* 62, 145, 1975.
7. **Basin, H. and Doria, G.,** The metabolism of different immunoglobulin classes in irradiated mice. III. Effects of supra-lethal doses of x-rays, *Int. J. Radiat. Biol.,* 17, 359, 1970.
8. **Carlson, D. E. and Gengozian, N.,** Radiation exposure-rate dependence of the immune response in mice, *Radiology,* 97, 433, 1970.
9. **Carlson, D. C. and Gengozian, N.,** The effect of acute radiation exposure rates on formation of hemagglutinating antibody in mice, *J. Immunol.,* 106, 1353, 1971.
10. **Carlson, D. C. and Lubet, R. A.,** Effects of sublethal gamma radiation on T and B cell activity in the antibody response of mice, *Radiat. Res.,* 65, 111, 1976.
11. **Gottlieb, C. F. and Gengozian, N.,** The humoral immune response in mice after neutron or x-irradiation at different dose rates, *J. Immunol.,* 109, 711, 1972.
12. **Gottlieb, C. F. and Gengozian, N.,** Radiation dose, dose rate, and quality in suppression of the humoral immune response, *J. Immunol.,* 109, 719, 1972.
13. **Hayakawa, J. and Tsuchiya, T.,** The long-term effect of single whole-body irradiation on graft-versus-host reactivity in mice in comparison with the effect of bone marrow reconstitution and of continuous irradiation, *Radiat. Res.,* 68, 31, 1976.
14. **Slavin, S., Strober, S., Fuks, Z., and Kaplan, H.,** Induction of specific tissue transplantation tolerance using fractionated total lymphoid irradiation in adult mice: long-term survival of allogenic bone marrow and skin grafts, *J. Exp. Med.,* 146, 34, 1977.
15. **Chanana, A. D., Cronkite, E. P., and Joel, D. D.,** Selective Immunosuppression by radiation, *Radiation and the Lymphatic System,* Ballou, J. E., Ed., ERDA Symp. Ser. 37, CONF-740930, National Technical Information Service, Springfield, Va., 153, 1976.
16. **Slavin, S., Strober, S., Fuks, Z., and Kaplan, H.,** Long term survival of skin allografts in mice treated with fractionated total lymphoid irradiation, *Science,* 193, 1252, 1976.
17. **Souto, J. and Anderson, D. L.,** Bone marrow changes following blood replacement from irradiated donors, *Trans. N.Y. Acad. Sci.,* Ser. II, 32(4), 441, 1970.
18. **Souto, J. and Anderson, D. L.,** Peripheral leukocyte changes in sheep after blood replacement from irradiated donors, *Trans. N.Y. Acad. Sci.,* Ser. II, 32(4), 428, 1970.

19. **Fuks, Z., Strober, S., Bobrove, A. M., Sasazuki, T., McMichael, A., and Kaplan, H. S.,** Long term effects of radiation on T and B lymphocytes in the peripheral blood of patients with Hodgkin's disease, *J. Clin. Invest.*, 58, 803, 1976.
20. **Birkeland, S. A., Moesner, J., Kalnaes, O., and Jensen, T. S.,** Endolymphatic irradiation with ^{198}Au and ^{32}P as immunosuppression in renal transplantation, *Radiat. Res.*, 65, 371, 1976.
21. **Nelson, D. F., Chaffey, J. T., and Hellman, S.,** The long term effects of x-irradiation on the ability of the spleen to support clonogenic proliferation, *Radiat. Res.*, 58, 497, 1974.
22. **Haran-Ghera, N., Lieberman, M., and Kaplan, H. S.,** Direct action of a leukemogenic virus on the thymus, *Cancer Res.*, 26, 438, 1966.
23. **Haran-Ghera, N. and Peled, A.,** The mechanism of radiation action in leukaemogenesis. Isolation of a leukaemogenic filterable agent from tissues of irradiated and normal C57BL mice, *Br. J. Cancer*, 21, 730, 1967.
24. **Haran-Ghera, N.,** The mechanism of radiation action in leukaemogenesis. The role of radiation in leukaemia development, *Br. J. Cancer*, 21, 739, 1967.
25. **Clapp, N. K. and Yuhas, J. M.,** Suggested correlation between radiation-induced immunosuppression and radiogenic leukemia virus, *J. Natl. Cancer Inst.*, 51, 1211, 1973.
26. **Peled, A. and Haran-Ghera, N.,** The cellular basis of immunosuppression caused by the radiation leukemia virus, *Immunology*, 26, 323, 1974.
27. **Ihle, J. N., McEwan, R., and Bengali, K.,** Radiation leukemia in C57Bl/6 mice. I. Lack of serological evidence for the role of endogenous ecotropic viruses in pathogenesis, *J. Exp. Med.*, 144, 1391, 1976.
28. **Schechmeister, I. L., Bond, V. P., and Swift, M. N.,** The susceptibility of irradiated mice to infection as a function of postirradiation time, *J. Immunol.*, 68, 87, 1952.
29. **Donaldson, D. M., Marcus, S., Gyi, K. K., and Perkins, E. H.,** The influence of immunization and total body x-irradiation in intracellular digestion by peritoneal phagocytes, *J. Immunol.*, 76, 192, 1965.
30. **Kornfield, L. and Miller, C. P.,** Restoration of serum bactericidal activity and prevention of its loss in x-irradiated mice, *J. Immunol.*, 86, 215, 1961.
31. **Singer, I.,** The effect of x-irradiation on infections with *Plasmodium berghei* in the white mouse, *J. Infect. Dis.*, 92, 97, 1953.
32. **Hotchin, J. and Weigand, H.,** The effects of pretreatment with x-rays on the pathogenesis of lymphocytic choriomeningitis in mice. I. Host survival, virus multiplication, and leukocytosis, *J. Immunol.*, 87, 675, 1961.
33. **Raff, M. C.,** T and B lymphocytes and immune responses, *Nature (London)*, 242, 19, 1973.
34. **Stockman, G. D., Gallagher, M. T., Heim. L. R., South, M. A., and Trentin, J. J.,** Differential stimulation of mouse lymphoid cells by phytohemagglutinin and pokeweed mitogen, *Proc. Soc. Exp. Biol. Med.*, 136, 980, 1971.
35. **Geha, R. S., Rosen, F. S., and Merler, E.,** Unresponsiveness of human B lymphocytes to phytohemagglutinin, *Nature (London)*, 248, 526, 1974.
36. **Facchini, A., Maraldi, N. M., Bartoli, S., Farulla, A., and Manzoli, F. A.,** Changes in membrane receptors of B and T human lymphocytes exposed to ^{60}Co gamma rays, *Radiat. Res.*, 68, 339, 1976.
37. **Reddy, M. M., Goh, K., and Hempelmann, L. H.,** B and T lymphocytes in man. I. Effect of infant thymic irradiation on the circulating B and T lymphocytes, *Radiation and the Lymphatic System*, Ballou, J. E., Ed., ERDA Symp. Ser. 37, CONF-74093O, National Technical Information Service, Springfield, Va., 192, 1976.
38. **Stjernswärd, J., Jondal, M., Vanky, F., Wigzell, H., and Sealy, R.,** Lymphopenia and change in distribution of human B and T lymphocytes in peripheral blood induced by irradiation for mammary carcinoma, *Lancet*, i, 1353, 1972.
39. **Byfield, P. E., Stratton, J. A., and Small, R.,** Lymphocyte response after radiotherapy, *Lancet*, 309, 1974.
40. **Han, T., Pauly, J., and Minowada, J.,** Differential effects of irradiation on cultured T and B lymphoid cells, *Blood*, 42, 1026, 1973.
41. **Kataoka, Y. and Sado, T.,** The radiosensitivity of T and B lymphocytes in mice, *Immunology*, 29, 121, 1975.
42. **Anderson, R. E., Sprent, J., and Miller, J. F. A. P.,** Cell-to-cell interaction in the immune response. VIII. Radiosensitivity of thymus derived lymphocytes, *J. Exp. Med.*, 135, 771, 1972.
43. **Tigelaar, R. E. and Asofsky, R.,** Synergy among lymphoid cells mediating the graft-versus-host response, *J. Exp. Med.*, 137, 239, 1973.
44. **Kadish, J. L. and Basch, R. S.,** Thymic regeneration after lethal irradiation: Evidence for an intra-thymic radioresistant T cell precursor, *J. Immunol.*, 114, 452, 1975.
45. **Kadish, J. L. and Basch, R. S.,** Hematopoietic thymocyte precursors. I. Assay and kinetics of the appearance of progeny, *J. Exp. Med.*, 143, 1082, 1976.

46. **Blomgren, H. and Andersson, B.,** Reappearance and relative importance of immunocompetent cells in the thymus, spleen and lymph nodes following lethal-x-irradiation and bone marrow reconstitution in mice, *J. Immunol.*, 106, 831, 1971.
47. **Blemgren, H. and Andersson, B.,** Evidence for a small pool of immunocompetent cells in the mouse thymus, *Exp. Cell. Res.*, 57, 185, 1969.
48. **Decleve, A., Gerber, G. B., Leonard, A., Lambert-Collier, M., Sassen, A., and Maisin, J. R.,** Regeneration of thymus, spleen and bone marrow in x-irradiated AKR mice, *Radiat. Res.*, 51, 318, 1972.
49. **Pettersen, E. O., Bøyum, A., and Laane, B. F. M.,** X-ray inactivation of murine bone marrow cells as measured by the spleen colony assay and the diffusion chamber technique, *Radiat. Res.*, 58, 409, 1974.
50. **Ito, T., Kino, T., and Cudkowicz, G.,** B-cell differentiation in the splenic environment: Acquired susceptibility to the helper function of irradiated T cells, *J. Immunol.*, 110, 596, 1973.
51. **Chanana, A. D., Grecher, G., Cronkite, E. P., Joel, D., and Schnappauf, Hp.,** The influence of extracorporeal irradiation of the blood and lymph on skin homograft rejection, *Radiat. Res.*, 27, 330, 1966.
52. **Chanana, A. D., Grecher, G., and Cronkite, E. P.,** Histologic observations on skin autografts, isografts and allografts in cattle, *Am. J. Pathol.*, 49, 1125, 1966.
53. **King, R., DeGiorgi, L. S., Royster, R. L., Wolf, J. S., and Levitt, S. H.,** Irradiation as an immunosuppressive agent in organ transplantation, *Radiology*, 93, 297, 1969.
54. **Gergely, N. F. and Coles, J. C.,** Prolongation of heterotopic cardiac allografts in dogs by topical radiation, *Transplantation*, 9, 193, 1970.
55. **Ford, W. L.,** The mechanism of lymphopenia produced by chronic irradiation of the rat spleen, *Br. J. Exp. Pathol.*, 49, 502, 1968.
56. **Yoshida, T., Hunter, R. L., and Benacerraf, B.,** Immunosuppressive effect of the depletion of circulating lymphocytes by chronic irradiation of the rat spleen, *J. Immunol.*, 101, 1111, 1970.
57. **Hollingsworth, J. W., Carr, J., and Ford, W. L.,** Lymphopenia produced by polythylene-^{32}P strips applied to the rabbit appendix, *Cell. Immunol.*, 4, 407, 1972.
58. **Eltringham, J. R. and Weissman, I.,** Regional lymph node irradiation: Effect on immune responses, *Radiology*, 94, 438, 1970.
59. **Visakorpi, R.,** The effect of irradiation on macrophage migration inhibition, *Immunology*, 27, 145, 1974.
60. **Song, C. W. and Levitt, S. H.,** Radiation effects on the formation of effector cells and on the cytotoxicity of the effector cells, *Radiation and the Lymphatic System*, Ballou, J. E., Ed., ERDA Symp. Ser. 37, CONF-740930, National Technical Information Service, Springfield, Va., 169, 1976.
61. **Stoner, R., Terres, G., Cottier, H., and Hess, M.,** Radiosensitivity of antibody responses and radioresistant secondary tetanus antitoxin responses, *Radiation and the Lymphatic System*, Ballou, J. E., Ed., ERDA Symp. Ser. 37, CONF-740930, National Technical Information Service, Springfield, Va., 175, 1976.
62. **Swasdikul, D. and Block, M.,** Effect of radiation upon the embryonic thymus, *Radiat. Res.*, 50, 73, 1972.
63. **Takada, Y. and Takada, A.,** Proliferation of donor hematopoietic cells in irradiated and unirradiated host mice, *Transplantation*, 12, 334, 1971.
64. **Kadish, J. L. and Basch, R. S.,** Hematopoietic thymocyte precursors, *J. Exp. Med.*, 143, 1082, 1976.

INDEX

A

B

C

D

E

F

G

H

I

J

K

L

M

N

R

S

T

U

V

W

X

Z